conquering heart attacks and strokes

conquering heart attacks and strokes

your 10 step self-defense plan

Reader's
Digest

Montreal • New York

about this book

If you're reading this page, you've already taken your first step toward protecting yourself and your family from a heart attack or stroke. You'll soon discover that *Conquering Heart Attacks & Strokes—Your 10 Step Self-Defense Plan* is clear and practical, giving you all the information you need to understand how problems arise, assess your own or a loved one's vulnerability and formulate a comprehensive strategy to fight back.

What's more, the advice in this book will help you to incorporate heart- and brain-protecting habits into everyday life in easily manageable steps. You'll learn how ingredients like a hearty breakfast, laughter, sunshine, dark chocolate, friendship and red wine are all part of the recipe for a long, healthy life. You'll be able to decide which tactics suit you best and, because the self-defense plan is easy to adopt and enjoyable to maintain, you'll be motivated to persevere, so that your strategy evolves into long-term protection.

how to use this book

If you prefer to browse through books instead of reading them all the way through, you'll find that each chapter here is self-contained, so that you can dip in to find information fast on any topic of particular concern—be it the symptoms of a stroke or the best way to lose weight, assessing your own risk factors or choosing heart-friendly foods.

Though each chapter can be read individually, together they build into a coherent step-by-step plan that you can easily tailor to your own risks and needs. Chapter 1 will enable you to understand just what you're dealing with: the widespread damage to arteries (the tiny tubes that carry blood around the body) that ultimately underpins most heart attacks and strokes, and the multiple factors that can affect your risk.

In chapter 2 you'll find out what happens during the course of a heart attack or a stroke and, most crucially, what actions to take. These events don't necessarily appear the way they're portrayed on television or in films, and it's surprising how many people simply don't recognize what's happening right away, delaying vital treatment for themselves or their loved ones.

Next, we suggest that you do the comprehensive self-assessment in chapter 3. This will enable you to discover the factors that may influence your individual risk, so that you are aware which of these you need to take action against. Then, in chapter 4, you'll be able to develop your own personalized plan to deal with your risks.

The subsequent chapters deal with specific areas of risk: your diet, weight, activity levels, environment and psychological factors. You'll know from your self-assessment which of these are most relevant for you, so you may want to concentrate on these first. But be sure to read all the chapters, because together they will undoubtedly help you build a unique and personal survival kit to defend yourself against both heart attacks and strokes. Then, in the last chapter, you'll learn how to keep your plan going to give you long-term protection for the rest of your life.

Contents

NOTE TO READERS

While the creators of this work have made every effort to be as accurate and up to date as possible, medical and pharmacological knowledge is constantly changing. Readers are recommended to consult a qualified medical specialist for individual advice. The writers, researchers, editors and publishers of this work cannot be held liable for any errors and omissions, or actions that may be taken as a consequence of information contained within this work.

introduction

While many people are aware of the dangers of heart attacks and strokes, relatively few realize that most of these events are, in essence, avoidable. Indeed, although both conditions now rank among the leading causes of death in most countries, at least 80 percent of premature deaths linked to heart disease and strokes could be prevented by adopting simple measures such as eating healthily, doing regular physical activity and avoiding tobacco, according to the World Health Organization. And as many as 90 percent of first heart attacks could be avoided by making similar lifestyle changes, according to the landmark Interheart study, which involved 15,000 people from 52 countries. In *Conquering Heart Attacks & Strokes—Your 10 Step Self-Defense Plan,* you'll discover simple ways to achieve these aims, and many more tactics that could dramatically reduce your personal risk.

Heart attacks and strokes are usually due to underlying cardiovascular disease, a condition featuring body-wide damage to the delicate lining of arteries, the tubes that carry oxygen and nutrient-rich blood to all the organs, tissues and cells in your body. You'll learn how the simple lifestyle changes you make to protect against heart attacks and strokes can dramatically cut your risk of many other conditions, too.

The advice in this book will help you to conquer linked problems such as obesity, high blood pressure, peripheral vascular disease and diabetes, and could also help you to reduce your risk of seemingly unrelated conditions such as arthritis, depression, osteoporosis and even cancer. It will help you to preserve your teeth, eyesight and hearing into old age, maintain strength, mobility and independence, and give you increased energy and joy in living.

DEFENSE AGAINST LIFESTYLE DISEASES

The same risk factors that can cause strokes and heart attacks are believed to underlie a host of other conditions. In fact, scientists are increasingly pinning a whole range of so-called lifestyle diseases on, well, our lifestyles: urbanized, stressed, sedentary and overfed but undernourished.

By targeting the root causes, the strategies described here offer you personal protection against these modern enemies. Not only will following the plan enhance the rest of your life, it will probably prolong it. Studies show that people who adopt these tactics are less likely to die prematurely from heart disease, stroke or from any cause. Cardiovascular disease is among the most deadly of the lifestyle diseases. Read on, and you'll understand the threat, learn how to respond to an attack and know just what you need to do to build up effective physical and mental defenses. You'll understand the damaging role that Western diets, inactivity, stress and related factors play in the development of these disorders. And you'll see that this is potentially good news, because such lifestyle elements are within everyone's power to change.

YOUR HEALTH, YOUR CHOICES

This is a book that encourages you to take positive action, rather than be a passive bystander to your own health, and to believe that heart disease and stroke can be beaten. It gives you all the information, tools and advice you need to combat cardiovascular disease in a coherent strategy that will enable you to take charge of your own health and to enjoy the benefits. Some goals may seem challenging, but there are plenty of tips, tricks and surprising suggestions to help you to stay with the plan and meet your targets.

Perhaps you've been told by your doctor that you have high blood pressure or high cholesterol and are at increased risk. Possibly you are aware that your lifestyle is less than healthy and are already feeling the effects. Perhaps a friend, parent or sibling has been affected, or you may even have already suffered an attack.

Whatever your reasons for reading this book, and whatever your current health status, you'll find that it is a highly effective field manual of all the essential information you need to recognize warning signs, know when to act and what to do, assess your own risk and minimize future threat. You'll also discover inspiring stories about people who have overcome cardiovascular conditions, spotted the symptoms and rescued a loved one or applied their skills to save a life. You'll gain understanding of the tactics you need to help yourself, as well as what medical input is required and when, and how the latest screening tests, drug treatments and surgical techniques can help.

CLEARING THE FOG OF MEDIA MESSAGES

The media constantly bombards us with messages about health. Television, newspapers, the Internet—they're all crammed with medical stories, statistics and advice. The trouble is, when it comes to cardiovascular disease, many of them are gloomy, pessimistic or negative. We're all too fat, our favorite foods are potentially toxic, the rates of diseases such as diabetes are rocketing, heart attacks kill you, strokes result in permanent disablement, you should avoid everything you like, stop smoking, eat more fiber, get more exercise … it's often so off-putting, that it's no wonder that many people simply tune out.

WHY THIS PLAN REALLY WORKS

Conquering Heart Attacks & Strokes—Your 10 Step Self-Defense Plan has a different approach because the starting point is you. While the risk of succumbing to a heart attack or a stroke is a serious concern, and the thought of these threats is genuinely frightening, the aim of this book is to explain and provide information and solutions that will allay your fears. It may seem at times that the outcome of serious medical events is out of our hands, but the sort of knowledge you'll find here can help you to take control of your own destiny.

You'll also discover that protecting your health doesn't have to require Herculean effort, constant self-denial and a punishing routine of intimidating, intensive cardiovascular workouts. This book doesn't plug some trendy diet, exercise craze or the latest wonder supplement. Instead, the advice spans the broad range of what today's medical experts now know about cardiovascular disease, and all the information is supported by authoritative medical facts and scientific studies. As well as explaining all the vital details that your doctor would tell you—if only he or she had all day to sit and talk about it—here you'll find information and advice that even your doctor may not be aware of. And you'll learn about the miracle tools that specialists can use to protect you, and how modern medicine can make a dramatic difference to your survival chances if you are threatened by stroke or heart attack.

FAR FROM INEVITABLE

The book's clear message is that cardiovascular disease is not an inevitable consequence of getting older. In fact, it's eminently preventable, as long as you are aware of the key facts and risks underlying most cardiovascular disease. Even though most people don't think much about these dangers until they get to a certain age, it's never too late to make positive changes.

Of course, there are certain risk factors that you cannot alter—your gender, genes and family history, for example. But, as you'll learn, there is so much that you can do to counteract these. And while some damage may have been done by past bad habits, research reveals that much of this may be undone by taking appropriate action now, whatever your age or current state of health. So here you'll find the low-down on tried and tested ways to halt the progress of cardiovascular disease, combat the underlying causes, cut risk factors and boost your protection.

How do you achieve all this? You probably know that good nutrition, an active lifestyle and avoiding smoking are crucial. The book doesn't preach. You won't be encouraged to live on brown rice and lettuce, pound the treadmill in the gym for hours each week (unless you want to) and drink nothing but water.

ENJOYING LIFE IS THE KEY

Instead, you'll discover how healthy living can be a joy. You'll find out why a glass of red wine with dinner and a square of luscious dark chocolate to follow can be a valid part of your defense plan. You'll learn about the heart-protecting effects of having fun, and why it is important to burn calories doing activities that you enjoy, whether it's singing, gardening or scuba diving. And how about the health benefits of watching a comedy film, chatting with friends or relaxing in the sunshine?

The message of *Conquering Heart Attacks & Strokes—Your 10 Step Self-Defense Plan* is that, whatever your risk (and almost everyone has some potential risk) you can reduce it and take charge of your health in a way that suits you. It's about making the most of everything modern medicine can offer while fighting these potential killers on your own terms. It's about enjoying life while empowering yourself to beat the threat of stroke and heart attack, recognising that the best person to protect you against disease, disability and premature death is you. And, finally, the advice in this book doesn't simply aim to help you avoid these conditions, prevent disability and prolong life, but also to ensure that all those extra years you stand to gain are as healthy and happy as they can possibly be.

—The Editors
Reader's Digest

self-defense plan
STEP
1

HEART ATTACKS AND STROKES CAN AFFECT ALMOST ANYONE, BUT THE GOOD NEWS IS THAT MOST OF THE CAUSES ARE PREVENTABLE. STEP 1 SETS OUT THE BATTLEGROUND—THE BUILDUP OF CONDITIONS THAT CAN PUT YOU AT RISK—AND REVEALS HOW A LITTLE KNOWLEDGE AND A FEW SIMPLE STRATEGIES ARE THE MOST POWERFUL DEFENSE.

Know what
you're up against

Every year, hundreds of thousands of North Americans suffer from a heart attack or stroke. Such events may seem to occur without warning but are almost always the result of underlying disorders. Plus, as you'll discover, they are far from inevitable if these conditions are prevented or treated in time.

Cardiovascular disease is the medical name for problems affecting the heart and blood vessels, which can so severely disrupt blood flow that a life-threatening heart attack or stroke occurs. Blood circulates constantly throughout the body, carrying to thousands of billions of cells the oxygen and the nutrients they need to survive. At the center of this vast and wonderful delivery system is the heart, a powerful pump that drives blood along a network of 60,000 miles (100,000 km) of blood vessels. Even when you are resting, it takes just over a minute for your blood to be pumped around your body.

But what happens if something obstructs the flow? Just as a car accident on a busy street may quickly lead to a serious pile-up, the consequences can be dangerous. The ten steps described in this book will help you to not only counteract most of the risks but also to improve your general health and boost your chances of a long, active and happy life.

LIFESTYLE CHANGES MAKE A DIFFERENCE

A wide range of factors contribute to the development of cardiovascular disease. Some, such as smoking, high blood pressure, lack of exercise and obesity, are well-known. You may also be aware that stress can contribute to the dangers of heart attacks and strokes, that people with diabetes are more at risk of heart disease, or that high cholesterol levels in the blood can "harden" arteries, narrowing them and increasing the chance of both heart attacks and strokes.

FRESH CHALLENGES

There are other, more surprising conditions associated with cardiovascular disease that medical studies have uncovered in recent years. Excess abdominal fat, for example, has been shown to be an important risk factor, while snoring and gum disease may also be linked. This book offers a wealth of advice on how to assess and deal with these associated conditions, as well as a host of tips to inspire you to make the long-lasting changes that will protect you throughout your life.

TACTICAL ADVANTAGE

If you are not sick right now, you may find it hard to believe that you are at risk. And research has shown that the younger you are, the less likely you are to accept that you could suffer from a heart attack or stroke. Doctors in Israel proved this point when they examined the medical records of 41,000 young people. They found that more than one in ten knew that they had a family history of cardiovascular disease, yet these people were no more likely to do exercise or avoid smoking than others with no genetic risk. Not only that, but they were more likely to be obese and have treatable conditions such as high blood pressure or high blood sugar.

Reading the information in this book will give you a vital tactical advantage. You will realize how much you can do to help yourself—even if you have a family history of cardiovascular problems. Then, as you spot risks that might affect you personally, such as high blood pressure, you will learn how you can adapt your everyday life to reduce them.

YOU ARE NOT ALONE

Just about everyone is vulnerable in some way, which is why cardiovascular disease is so potentially dangerous. But most of us can take

troubleshooting Q&A

My uncle had a heart attack in his fifties. Am I at risk too?

Having a family history of heart disease does statistically increase your risk of developing a problem yourself, and the closer the relative, the higher the risk. Tell your doctor, and arrange to get your cholesterol and blood pressure checked regularly. And read on. You can't change your family history, but, as you'll discover, healthy lifestyle measures can substantially reduce your risk.

an amazing transport system

Your blood travels thousands of miles around your body carrying the oxygen and nutrients that you need to survive. The heart plays a central role, pumping out the oxygen-rich blood it receives from the lungs into arteries, which deliver it to thousands of billions of cells, and simultaneously pumping blood back through veins to the lungs to receive a fresh load of oxygen. The clearer your arteries, the more efficient the system.

Blood vessels supplying the head and neck include the carotid artery. The brain uses about 20 percent of the body's blood and needs 25 percent of the body's oxygen to function at its best.

Figure-eight circulation

Having two separate circulation routes that meet in the heart means that your tissues receive only oxygen-rich blood.

Oxygen-enriched blood travels from the lungs to the heart, which drives it out to the rest of the body.

The aorta is the largest and most important artery of the body. It stretches from the heart to the lower abdomen and carries oxygenated blood under high pressure.

Deoxygenated blood from the body returns to the heart, which pumps it to the lungs for a fresh load of oxygen.

The pulmonary circulation goes through your lungs.

Your legs are supplied with a massive network of arteries and veins. Keeping active helps to ensure that they remain clear and transport blood effectively to the muscles and other tissues.

The systemic circulation goes through the rest of your body.

some action to reduce that risk. As scientists understand more and more about how cardiovascular disease develops, one thing has become crystal clear: The way you live plays an important role. This book will give you the tools not only to reduce your risk, but also to reverse some of the damage that may already have occurred inside your arteries.

IT'S ALL ABOUT LIFESTYLE

Medical research indicates that lifestyle plays a huge role in determining an individual's likelihood of developing heart disease, and there are many small adjustments that can dramatically improve your cardiovascular health. And this doesn't mean giving up all the little pleasures that make life worthwhile; defending yourself does not need to be about self-denial.

You will discover how sensuous pleasures, such as consuming red wine or dark chocolate, getting a massage or laughing with friends, can actually aid you in the fight. *Conquering Heart Attacks & Strokes* will show you how to incorporate these defense strategies into everyday living. As a bonus, they'll also improve your general health.

what causes the problem?

To reduce your risk of suffering from a heart attack or stroke, it's worth trying to understand how and why cardiovascular disease occurs. It starts in a small way, with tiny changes in the walls of arteries that set off a process that makes fats called lipids—together with cholesterol, calcium and other substances in the blood—get sucked into the arterial lining.

Gradually these fatty deposits build up and cause a narrowing of the inside of the arteries, which in turn restricts blood flow. At the same time, the deposits may harden, making the walls of the arteries thicker and less flexible, so that they are less able to expand and contract to regulate blood flow. That means that when you run, for example, your arteries are unable to widen to allow more oxygen-rich blood to flow to the muscles. You may find that you get out of breath quickly or start to experience chest pains.

The medical term for this is atherosclerosis—although it is frequently described as "hardening" of the arteries—and the substance that adheres to the arterial walls is called plaque. A buildup of plaque inside the

nine everyday changes that could save your life

No matter where you live, and no matter what your age or gender, the findings of a landmark medical study published in 2004 hold an important message for everyone: a great deal of cardiovascular disease is preventable because most of its causes are linked to the way we live.

Known as the Interheart study, this worldwide examination of risk factors for heart disease provides compelling evidence that the daily lifestyle choices made by individuals can improve the health of their arteries and reduce their risk of heart attacks and strokes. More than 15,000 men and women from 52 countries took part in the study. All had one thing in common: they had experienced their first heart attacks. Participants were questioned about the details of their lifestyles, medical and family histories and personal circumstances. They were given a physical examination, blood samples were taken, and they had their waist and hip circumferences measured. The results were then compared with those from healthy people living in the same communities.

When scientists analysed the mountain of data generated by the study, they came up with a startling finding: just nine factors accounted for 90 percent of all first-time heart attacks. The study made it clear that, while rates of cardiovascular disease vary from country to country, in almost every geographic region, men and women of all ages and ethnic backgrounds are vulnerable for the same nine reasons.

On the basis of such research, the Heart and Stroke Foundation of Canada and the American Heart Association insist that death from coronary artery disease—which claims nearly one in three lives in North America—is largely preventable. The message from Interheart is clear: Change your lifestyle and live longer.

the interheart 9

Each one of the nine risk factors identified by the Interheart study suggest that cardiovascular disease is far from inevitable. Each one is linked to unhealthy lifestyle choices, which can—with a few everyday changes—be modified to reduce your risk of both heart attacks and strokes.

1 Abnormal blood fats

2 Smoking

3 High blood pressure

4 Diabetes

5 Stress

6 Obesity, especially abdominal fat

7 Eating too few fruits and vegetables

8 A lack of daily exercise

9 Excess alcohol intake

the cholesterol story

You hear a lot about cholesterol, and it does play a significant role in the health of your heart and circulatory system. Cholesterol in the blood takes the form of small packages called lipoproteins, made up of lipids (fats) and protein. There are two kinds in your bloodstream: "bad" LDL (low-density lipoprotein) cholesterol and "good" HDL (high-density lipoprotein) cholesterol. Too much LDL—often the result of eating a diet high in saturated fats—increases the risk of atherosclerosis, the narrowing of the arteries that can lead to heart attacks and strokes. But HDL carries LDL cholesterol back to the liver for reprocessing and actually protects the heart.

If you have a high level of LDL cholesterol in your blood, the low-density lipoproteins can begin to adhere to the artery walls. This buildup contributes to the formation of plaque, which makes arteries narrower so blood cannot easily pass through to supply oxygen and nutrients. This sticky plaque then attracts even more plaque, and a vicious circle begins.

coronary arteries that supply blood to the muscle of the heart is a cardiovascular condition known as coronary artery disease. The narrowed arteries cannot supply sufficient oxygen-rich blood to the heart muscle to cope with periods of higher demand, such as during exercise.

CHEST PAIN

One common symptom of coronary artery disease is pain or discomfort in the chest, known as angina. It can be brought on by physical activity, cold weather, intense emotions such as anger or even a heavy meal. Angina indicates that, at times of increased demand, your heart is desperately craving a better blood supply.

The symptoms are not unlike a muscle cramp after undertaking exercise, though the sensation of heaviness or tightness in your chest may spread to your arms, neck, jaw, back or stomach. The discomfort usually subsides within minutes and won't cause any permanent damage to your heart. But it is an important wake-up call. You should consult your doctor and consider how your diet and lifestyle might be affecting your health.

If the pain suddenly gets worse or occurs when you haven't exerted yourself and is not relieved by rest or medication, seek urgent medical help. Doctors call this "unstable angina" and it can be caused by a small blood clot partially blocking a coronary artery. Unstable angina is very dangerous and indicates a much higher risk of a full-blown heart attack.

a heart crisis

The most common cause of a heart attack is a blood clot that completely blocks a coronary artery, cutting off blood supply to the heart.

Scientists now know that so-called "soft" plaque can be the dangerous trigger. Hard plaque contains more calcium and can grow relatively large, narrowing arteries, restricting blood flow and causing chest pain or high blood pressure. By contrast, "soft" plaque, which causes less narrowing but is loaded with fatty deposits, can easily rupture without warning.

A rupture causes the lipids (blood fats) and other debris to spill out from the artery wall and form a clot which could block vital blood flow to an area of the heart muscle. The rupture of soft plaque is thought to be responsible for about 85 percent of all heart attacks. Patches of soft plaque are also more difficult to detect because standard tests, such as CT scans, tend to measure calcium deposits, a sign of hard plaque.

OTHER CAUSES

While clots are the most common cause, a heart attack can also occur if an artery goes into spasm, temporarily stopping the flow of blood. Atherosclerosis (narrowing of the arteries) can cause such a spasm, or it can be a reaction to drugs such as amphetamines or cocaine, viral infection or smoking (particularly in women who also take birth control pills)—even stress.

PEOPLE WITH HEART DISEASE SHOULD TAKE LIFE EASY

Whether you suffer from angina or have had a heart attack or heart surgery, regular exercise is the best way to strengthen your heart muscle. Exercise helps to control blood pressure, cholesterol, weight gain and diabetes, and that usually means less medication. Crucially, exercise will reduce your risk of another attack.

When the explorer Sir Ranulph Fiennes had a massive heart attack in 2003, he was rushed to hospital for double bypass surgery. A few weeks later, he found that simply walking a few steps uphill made him breathless.
He kept at it. From walking, he progressed to jogging. Just four months later, Fiennes ran seven marathons on seven continents in seven days to raise money for the British Heart Foundation. In May 2009, at age 65, he conquered Mount Everest—one of the oldest people ever to reach the summit.

That's extraordinary, but anyone with heart disease can exercise. Just start slow and build it up gradually. In Step 7, you will learn how.

Less common causes of heart attacks include:

● Clots or other "debris" that travel from elsewhere in the body to lodge inside a coronary artery, a process known as coronary embolism.

● Clots that result from trauma following an accident, or conditions in which blood thickens and clots more easily—including, rarely, use of birth control pills in women.

● Congenital abnormalities of the coronary arteries, present since birth.

● Certain rare conditions, such as thrombocytosis, where the "stickiness" of the blood is increased, which can impede its flow and cause clots to form.

WEAKENING THE WALLS

Atherosclerosis can cause other problems, too. The plaque buildup may weaken arterial walls, causing a swelling called an aneurysm. The intense pressure of blood flowing through the artery can cause the arterial wall to balloon out and, in extreme cases, to burst.

A family history of aneurysms raises the risk, as does smoking and high blood pressure. The most common site for an aneurysm is the aorta, the largest artery, which carries blood down from the heart to the rest of the body. Without urgent treatment, a ruptured abdominal aortic aneurysm could be fatal.

Blocked arteries in other parts of the body may cause pain and a variety of other damaging effects. They can even result in disorders as serious as gangrene, when tissue dies because it is starved of blood.

CHILDHOOD CONCERNS

These problems are not only affecting older people. In recent studies, fatty streaks on the inside of artery walls have been found in youngsters, too—a development that worries scientists and health professionals. In a study of 294 adolescents at the Institute of Child Health in the United Kingdom, researchers noted blood vessel changes in teenagers as young as 13, whose artery walls were already losing their

SECRETweapon

PULSE CHECK

For good reason, some experts compare aneurysms to ticking time bombs: you get very little warning before a blood vessel bursts. However, there is one telling symptom of an abdominal aortic aneurysm (AAA), the most common type: Watch out for a pulsating sensation in the abdominal area, that is frequently accompanied by lower back pain.

But there is method of screening for AAA with ultrasound, and you shouldn't wait for symptoms before acting. The basic fact is that screening can be a lifesaver.

Older men are particularly at risk of AAA, so it's a good idea for all men over 60 who have smoked at any time in their lives to undergo the ultrasound AAA test. Fortunately, you only need to be screened once.

crucial elasticity.

The risk factors in children are the same as they are for adults: abnormal blood fats, high blood pressure, obesity and diabetes. In fact, the evidence that atherosclerosis can begin early in life is so powerful that doctors are being urged to take an active role in its prevention, by encouraging overweight children to modify their diet and do more exercise. Experts suggest that children between the ages of 2 and 5 consume low-fat dairy foods. Children 2 and younger should get full-fat milk and dairy, while skim milk and fat-free dairy should be fine for most kids over the age of 5.

THE FOOD SOLUTION

Stopping the flow of harmful fats circulating in your bloodstream will help to keep your arteries clear and plaque-free, whatever your age. That means adjusting your diet in such a way that you avoid saturated fats and reduce your LDL cholesterol levels (see page 18). The most effective dietary changes you can make are explained in Step 5.

Teenagers are being encouraged to eat more healthily in order to protect themselves against future problems.

Continued on p. 24 ▶

your body: under attack

When you think of inflammation, you may visualize a hot, red, tender area of skin – a site where your immune system is mounting a heated and healing defense against attack, which happens when a cut becomes infected. In much the same way, our immune system is programmed to react against what it sees as microbial invaders in our arteries. Scientists are discovering more about the key role played by this internal "inflammation" in the artery-damaging process called atherosclerosis.

Medical researchers no longer believe that high blood cholesterol is the only culprit in atherosclerosis, the process where fat-laden plaque is deposited on arterial linings. Most experts now acknowledge that the whole process of arterial damage is set off and sustained by inflammation.

What happens is that white blood cells—the frontline troops in our body's immune system—are attracted by the sludge-like plaque deposits inside artery walls. They bombard these deposits with chemicals, which in turn helps to create more plaque and prompts it to rupture, causing the formation of blood clots and leading to heart attacks. At high levels, inflammation can double or even quadruple the risk of heart attacks.

The theory of this inflammation "cascade" fits well with research showing that many of the traditional risk factors linked to heart attacks and strokes, such as high blood cholesterol levels, high blood pressure, diabetes and obesity, are factors that also provoke inflammation.

INFLAMMATION DETECTORS

Doctors hope to use this new understanding of how inflammation underlies atherosclerosis in order to predict the risk of heart attacks and strokes much earlier than was possible in the past. Several chemicals found in the bloodstream act as "markers" of inflammation in the body. One of these, known as CRP (C-reactive protein), increases when inflammation is present and can be valuable in monitoring disease activity. Increased CRP levels have also been linked with other cardiovascular risk factors, such as

REDalert !

FAT AND UNFIT?

Obesity increases the risk of inflammation, according to a study of 452 men published in the *British Journal of Sports Medicine*. The study found that white-blood-cell counts were lowest in men who were physically fit and highest in those who were most overweight. On average, the higher a man's proportion of body fat, the higher his white-cell count, supporting evidence that fat cells actually produce inflammatory chemicals. The researchers also noted that being fit seemed to counteract the effect of extra fat, suggesting that physical fitness plays a large role in combating inflammation.

smoking, high cholesterol and abdominal obesity. On the other hand, eating plenty of fish and having higher levels of vitamin C have been linked with lower CRP levels. (The role of key protective foods is discussed in Step 5.)

SENSITIVE BLOOD TEST

Recently, a new way of measuring inflammation related more specifically to the risk of heart disease has been developed, known as a high-sensitivity CRP test, or hsCRP. Research has shown that hsCRP levels are elevated years in advance of an individual's first heart attack or ischemic stroke, and raised levels are highly predictive of recurrent heart attacks and strokes, diabetes and death from cardiovascular disease. Cardiologists already use hsCRP as part of a combined test—which also measures levels of cholesterol and the blood fats known as triglycerides—to give the clearest profile yet of cardiovascular risk. Ask your doctor about whether you should have a CRP test done.

Keeping fit greatly reduces your risk of the type of inflammation that sparks off arterial damage.

stroke is a **brain attack**

Atherosclerosis can affect all arteries in the body, so it is not only your heart that could suffer damage. When plaque builds up on the carotid arteries supplying blood to the brain, narrowing the vessels and restricting blood flow, it is known as cerebrovascular disease. While there is no brain equivalent of angina—you won't get a headache, for instance—the blood flow to your brain is generally lowered, and less oxygen and fewer nutrients may get through to critical areas.

This is thought to be one of the reasons why older people may complain that they can't think clearly; they become more forgetful, for example, and have trouble concentrating and processing ideas as fast as they once could. Significantly, this is especially true of people who have been diagnosed with high blood pressure or cardiovascular disease.

WHAT TYPE OF STROKE?

Strokes are more complicated than heart attacks. The majority are called ischemic strokes and are caused by a clot blocking a blood vessel that has been narrowed by atherosclerosis. The clot may have formed following a rupture of plaque, which happens in the most common form of heart attack (see page 19), or it may have traveled from the heart, one of the arteries in the neck or elsewhere in the body. Clots that move through the bloodstream this way are known as emboli, and when they lodge in the brain the event is called a cerebral embolism.

However, around one in five strokes is due to bleeding in the brain following the tearing of an artery wall. This is known as a hemorrhagic stroke and is particularly likely to occur in an individual with high blood pressure. The effects of a hemorrhagic stroke are often more severe than those of ischemic strokes, and the treatments for the two types of strokes are very different, as explained on page 54.

identifying the triggers

Both heart attacks and strokes are generally the result of atherosclerosis that has built up over decades, but the culmination of this process in a sudden attack is often preceded by an event known as a trigger.

Triggers have one thing in common: They prompt the nervous system to flood the body with stress hormones, putting strain on the heart and blood vessels. A trigger factor can result in a sudden surge in blood pressure or make the heart beat faster—occasionally beyond the point at

I use birth control pills. Does this make me more at risk?

Probably not much, if at all. Very early types of contraceptive pill contained high doses of estrogen that could increase the risk of blood clots, and some studies suggested that older women who took the pill in its early days had a slightly increased risk of cardiovascular disease – but only while taking it. The hormone doses now used in the pill are much lower, and don't seem to increase the risk of heart attacks in young women with no other risk factors (such as smoking, diabetes or high blood pressure). And although the Pill does increase the chance of having a stroke, the risk is tiny – about 1 in 24,000 per year among women taking the Pill who don't smoke and have normal blood pressure. That's less than the risk of being killed in a road accident.

However, women who've had blood clots or strokes, who are 35 or older and smoke, have a history of estrogen-dependent cancer or have active liver diseaser or undiagnosed abnormal uterine bleeding shouldn't use estrogen-based contraception.

which it is able to cope with the extra workload. Some triggers narrow blood vessels, prompt clots to form or increase damage to the lining of arterial walls. Others may lead to a tear in a blood vessel or an erratic heart rhythm that may cause the heart to stop altogether.

Later in this book you will discover more about risk elements and the steps you can take to halt, and even reverse, the process of atherosclerosis. You will also learn about a whole range of factors that can trigger a heart attack or stroke—ranging from a powerful emotion such as anger, to a fat-laden meal or a bitterly cold day.

REDalert

MINI-STROKES

A transient ischemic attack (TIA), or mini-stroke, occurs if an artery supplying part of the brain becomes temporarily blocked, shutting off the blood supply. Any effects—such as slurred speech or a drooping facial muscle—are usually over in minutes, leaving no apparent damage, but may last as long as 24 hours.

However short-lived, a TIA should never be ignored, given that you run a 10 percent risk of a full-blown stroke in the week following a transient iscemic attack. Even if symptoms appear to go away, it is important to seek medical help immediately.

To picture the effects of high blood pressure, think of a river forced into a narrow gorge: your blood hurtles against the walls of narrowing arteries, damaging the inner lining.

silent enemy

High blood pressure is the main risk factor for strokes and a major risk factor for heart disease. If you have high blood pressure, you are three times more likely to develop heart disease or strokes—and twice as likely to die from one of those conditions—as people with lower levels.

Blood pressure is the force of blood flowing through your arteries and pushing against their vessel walls. You need some pressure to keep blood moving, but if the pressure is too high, the effect of blood pounding through the vessels thickens and hardens the arterial muscles, damaging the arteries' inner lining. Blood cells and fat deposits gather at the damaged areas, forming plaque. The consequence is a rapid acceleration in the hardening of the arteries.

Know your numbers

When did you last get your blood pressure checked? If you can't remember, make an appointment with your doctor today. One in three people with high blood pressure don't know they have it; there are no obvious symptoms. People with high blood pressure run about twice the lifetime risk of strokes as those with normal blood pressure, while hypertension is linked with a shorter life expectancy and greater risk of cardiovascular disease. Thousands of lives a year could be saved if more people were aware of their blood pressure and got treatment to bring their levels down.

When your blood pressure is measured, two readings are taken, expressed as an upper and a lower number. The upper number denotes systolic blood pressure, or the force on the artery walls when your heart is contracting to pump out blood. The lower number is the diastolic pressure, or the force when the heart is at rest between beats.

- A healthy reading is 120/80 or less (systolic pressure/diastolic pressure).
- A consistent reading of 140/90 or higher is diagnosed as high blood pressure, at any age, and requires treatment.

Blood pressure is measured in millimeters of mercury (mmHg). If your blood pressure is on the high side, a reduction of just 10mmHg in systolic pressure and 5mmHg in diastolic pressure will cut your risk of strokes by 38 percent, with a 16 percent risk reduction of heart disease.

working out your
personal risk

The nine risk factors identified by the worldwide Interheart study (see page 17) demonstrate that lifestyle is a major influence on cardiovascular health—and, by extension, that there are many things we can do to promote our own well-being. But they don't represent the full picture.

While lifestyle adjustments may have a beneficial effect on such factors as high blood pressure, high cholesterol, gum disease and obesity, there are a few things you cannot control, such as your age, gender and whether you have a family history of cardiovascular problems. And the study doesn't mention your emotional state, which can play a role, too. Stress, loneliness, a lack of outside interests, pessimism and anger are all negative factors that— together with other risks—may make you more vulnerable. Then there are also environmental factors such as air pollution, extremes of cold or heat, excessive noise and toxic chemicals.

REDalert

PLAYOFF WARNING

Calm down! Getting distraught while watching your favorite sports team lose a crucial match could trigger a heart attack. In the three days after the English soccer team lost to Argentina in a penalty shoot-out during the 1998 World Cup, hospital admissions for heart attacks in England soared by 25 percent. An earlier study in the Netherlands revealed a 50 percent increase in deaths from both heart attacks and strokes on the day the Dutch team was eliminated from the European soccer championship. There is one small consolation for female soccer fans: It was only men who were affected.

POSITIVE INTERVENTION

As doctors become better at identifying those patients most at risk from heart disease and strokes, they will be better able to pinpoint the most effective preventive treatments. For example, they may give statins (cholesterol-lowering drugs which also lower inflammation) to those with a raised level of the inflammation-detecting protein CRP (see pages 22–23), irrespective of their blood cholesterol level. Since about half of all strokes and heart attacks occur in people with a normal blood cholesterol level, this is potentially very important. And, in one review involving 2,557 people monitored for an average of eight years, people with raised CRP levels ran twice the risk of a heart attack or stroke even after taking account of other known risk factors.

Increased understanding of the inflammation "cascade" caused by the presence of plaque in the arteries (see page 22) also offers the prospect of better preventive treatment. Such treatment would be specifically

GET MOVING

Appropriate exercise can do much to prevent, counteract or reverse the internal changes that underlie cardiovascular disease. In fact, physical activity can have such beneficial effects on circulatory problems associated with diabetes and high blood pressure that, in some cases, it is possible for people who take up an exercise program to reduce their medication or even stop taking pills altogether.

Exercise may help to ward off strokes as well. A study looking at the benefits of exercise in people aged 50 to 77 who were suffering from depression demonstrated that, after 16 weeks of exercise, participants displayed sharper memories and better planning and organizational skills—a result of the improved flow of oxygen-rich blood to the brain. The results suggest that exercise might be able to offset some of the decline in mental acuity linked to the aging process.

Statins are often prescribed for people at high risk of heart disease to reduce "harmful" LDL cholesterol levels.

aimed at blocking this chain of events before it starts or interrupting its progress. For example, many people at high risk of developing cardiovascular disease are prescribed statins to reduce their level of LDL cholesterol. But statins are also anti-inflammatory, and research now shows that they can reduce the additional cardiovascular risk linked with raised CRP levels.

taking **the tests**

If you are experiencing symptoms such as chest pain or breathlessness that suggest a heart risk, your doctor may refer you for assessment by a specialist. The exploratory tests that could be offered include:

● **Electrocardiogram** (ECG or EKG)—a recording of the electrical activity of your heart. This may be done while you are lying down or, if you get symptoms predominantly after exertion, while you exercise on a treadmill. Sometimes you will be fitted with wires to monitor the electrical activity of your heart during a 24-hour period.

● **Magnetic Resonance Imaging** (MRI)—a scan that uses a very powerful magnet to create cross-section images of internal body tissues so doctors can see the physical structure of the heart. You will be asked to lie very still on the machine couch, which slides into the tunnel-like scanner. You may be offered headphones or ear plugs as the scanner is operating because, although painless, it is very noisy.

● **Radionuclide scans**—various tests in which tiny amounts of radioactive substances are injected into your bloodstream. When these reach the heart, they can be detected by a special camera, producing images of your coronary arteries or showing how well your heart is pumping. For one of these tests, myocardial perfusion imaging (MPI), an isotope injection is given after the patient has been pedaling on an exercise bike or treadmill. A scan is then performed to show the blood flow in the heart muscle.

● **Computed Tomography** (CT)—a special type of X-ray that produces detailed pictures of cross sections of the body. Sometimes it is used to assess how much calcium has been deposited in your coronary arteries—a measure of hard plaque, which is made up of calcium and collagen.

● **Angiography**—X-ray pictures taken after the injection of a special dye to reveal the coronary arteries.

If exploratory tests reveal that you have severe coronary artery disease, your doctor may recommend surgical treatment to reduce the risk of a heart attack. For example, it may be possible to open up the coronary arteries (angioplasty) or to bypass them altogether (coronary artery bypass graft surgery). You can find out more about these treatments in Step 2.

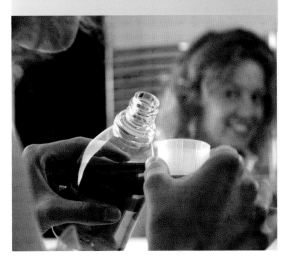

SECRETweapon

DENTAL HYGIENE

Gum disease has been linked with an increased risk of cardiovascular disease. Regular tooth-brushing and flossing will keep your gums healthy, and you should visit your dentist regularly for checkups. It is especially important to see your dentist if you have any bleeding from the gums. Using mouthwash daily also helps to kill off the bacteria that cause inflamed gums and can help to prevent the buildup of dental plaque, which leads to gum problems. See Step 8 for more details.

Continued on p32 ▶

hidden dangers of diabetes

The number of people diagnosed with diabetes – a risk factor for cardiovascular disease – is growing at an unprecedented rate. Experts link the increase to obesity.

Between 1980 and 2007, the percent of Americans diagnosed with diabetes increased 136 percent. In 2007, about 6 percent of the population had been diagnosed with the disease. Also, an estimated 9 million Canadians have diabetes or prediabetes; Canadian health-care costs are expected to hit or exceed $16.9 billion a year by 2030. In addition, millions more may have the condition and not know it. The bad news is that people with diabetes are up to eight times more likely than non-diabetics to die from cardiovascular disease.

There are two main types of diabetes mellitus: Type 1, which typically develops in childhood, and Type 2, which is by far the most common and largely responsible for the current explosion of diabetes cases. Both involve the action of insulin, a hormone produced by the pancreas, which promotes the uptake of glucose (sugar)—the body's main source of energy—into cells. Any upset in this function can lead to abnormally high levels of glucose in the blood, which causes problems and defects in various parts of the body.

While Type 1 is caused by the loss of insulin-producing cells and requires lifelong insulin treatment, Type 2, which tends to develop later in life—but is now being seen younger and younger—occurs either because the body isn't making sufficient insulin, or because cells have become resistant to its effects (insulin resistance). That means the body can't metabolize glucose properly (glucose intolerance). As a result, a dangerous vicious circle develops: Blood glucose levels rise and the body produces more insulin to lower them but, because the cells aren't responding properly, glucose continues to build up in the blood and the demand for insulin increases.

A CLUSTER OF RISK FACTORS

If you already have insulin resistance and glucose intolerance, studies show that you are likely to develop Type 2 diabetes within ten years unless you take some remedial action. While some of the risk may be inherited, weight gain and an inactive lifestyle intensify the problem.

Medical experts call the cluster of risk factors for both diabetes and cardiovascular problems "metabolic syndrome." The key features that they have identified include not only

---

REDalert !

TUMMY FAT DANGER

Abdominal fat releases lipids that are carried in the blood to the liver, where they may accumulate as a type of fat called triglycerides. Raised blood levels of triglycerides are linked with an increased risk of cardiovascular disease. In the liver, these fats can also disrupt the organ's key role in processing glucose (sugar) and insulin. Research has shown that the flow of lipids to the liver is greatest overnight and that this increases the risk of insulin resistance—partly explaining why people with large amounts of abdominal fat are at an increased risk of diabetes.

Research suggests that
losing just 5 to 7 percent of your body weight
can cut your risk of developing diabetes by 60 percent.

insulin resistance and glucose intolerance, but also abdominal obesity, high blood pressure, blood fat abnormalities and overly high levels of blood glucose. The condition is also linked to inflammation (see page 22) and blood clots. Studying this syndrome has helped doctors to understand how these conditions together cause underlying changes that contribute to cardiovascular disease and, ultimately, to your risk of heart attacks and strokes.

inside information

In one study of people in their sixties or older who had metabolic syndrome, the majority of those who followed a specific diabetes prevention program which included dietary and exercise recommendations regained normal blood glucose levels and reduced their risk factors for heart disease. On average, they lowered their chance of developing diabetes by 70 percent. By contrast, other people in the study, who only took medication specifically designed to reduce the chance of their developing diabetes, cut their risk by just 31 percent.

REDUCING THE RISK

While it is difficult to measure insulin levels directly, your doctor can use two simple glucose tests to assess whether you are glucose intolerant (and therefore likely to be insulin resistant). If the result of either test is abnormal, your doctor may well advise you to adopt the sort of lifestyle changes recommended in this book—by, for example, cutting your intake of calories and saturated (animal) fats by substituting lean chicken and fish for red meats and eating more fruit and vegetables. Boosting the amount of physical activity you undertake—an ideal level is 30–40 minutes brisk walking, at least five days a week— also increases the sensitivity of muscle cells to insulin, helping them to metabolize glucose. Research suggests that losing just 5 to 7 percent of your body weight can cut your risk of developing diabetes by 60 percent.

emerging evidence

Cardiovascular disease is not a clear-cut problem. It is caused by a web of factors, so scientific researchers are always searching for links to help them to discover precisely how and why it develops. All the following elements are thought to be significant:

- **Fat cells**—these normally act as energy storage, pumping out "fuel" in the form of fatty acids when the body calls for it. But fat tissue also produces hormones that regulate body weight. If you are overweight, it releases inflammatory chemicals too, which are thought to promote some of the complications linked with obesity, such as insulin resistance, diabetes, heart disease and arthritis.

- **Fibrinogen**—this protein produced by the liver is important in blood clotting. Raised fibrinogen levels are linked with inflammation and are found in people with insulin resistance and those who have suffered from coronary artery disease, heart attacks or strokes. It has been suggested that, as well as acting as a marker of risk, fibrinogen may contribute to the development of atherosclerosis.

- **Apolipoprotein B**—this protein, known as apoB, plays a key role in the production of cholesterol and its transport around the body. It bonds with LDL ("bad") cholesterol in the bloodstream. Raised apoB levels are associated with inflammation, and research shows that apoB is a better predictor of cardiovascular risk—and of how well an individual will respond to cholesterol-lowering drugs—than tests that simply measure cholesterol levels.

- **Homocysteine**—high levels of this blood protein have been linked to increased risk of high blood pressure and heart disease. Homocysteine is believed to damage cells that line the coronary arteries. While homocysteine levels can be reduced by taking folate, a vitamin found in raw fruit and vegetables, and antioxidant vitamins such as vitamin C, experts are still not sure if doing so directly reduces cardiovascular risk.

fighting back

Doctors now realize that cardiovascular disease is far more complicated than we once thought, and that there is a multitude of interlinked elements that may affect an individual's risk. Far too often, cardiovascular disease is diagnosed only after someone has experienced a heart attack or stroke. The plain fact is that you may have atherosclerosis and not know it. That is why it is so important to be aware of the risk factors and to take action before a dramatic event occurs.

DRAWING UP A STRATEGY

Your first line of defense against heart attacks and strokes is to identify your own personal risk factors and to develop a strategy to counteract them. The next step is to carry the strategy through. As you will discover,

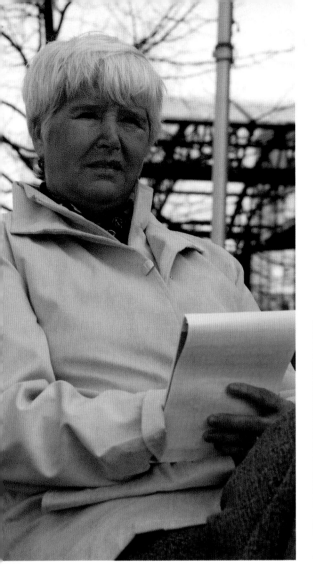

It's important to recognize your personal risk factors. Then you can draw up a practical plan to overcome and eliminate them – one by one.

making some small but crucial changes is not particularly difficult. Later steps in this book describe the easiest and simplest ways to influence those risks for the better and how to fit your control strategy into your daily routine, with accompanying tips to make the whole process more fun.

START NOW – TODAY

Look back—right now—at those nine factors identified by the Interheart study (page 17), and take note of how many of them apply, or might apply, to you. What could you do at this very moment to start to reduce your risk and to begin the push towards healthier arteries? Give up the next cigarette? Eat a piece of fruit? Go for a brisk walk?

One of the central messages of this book is that change is easiest and most effective if you make it in small stages. Think of it as a journey to a place you would really like to visit. You can't arrive instantly: Traveling

HAPPINESS

It's no joke, say scientists. Laughter and feel-good emotions can help to protect us from heart disease. Researchers at the University of Maryland School of Medicine found that, when we chuckle, the tissue that forms the inner lining of our blood vessels expands—a healthy response which increases blood flow. By contrast, mental stress caused blood vessels to constrict.

Listening to enjoyable music also increases blood flow to the arteries. Researchers believe that, when we experience pleasure, our brains release beneficial endorphins that directly affect our vascular system.

takes time. But each step you make will bring you a little closer to your destination. You will find out that each stage of the voyage can be a joy in itself, and the things you learn on the way will stay with you for ever.

SETTING GOALS

This book provides a great deal of advice and a wealth of practical tips for making vital lifestyle changes that can diminish your risk of diabetes, cardiovascular disease, heart attacks and strokes. But everyone needs to start by setting goals. For instance, if you are overweight, here are some goals you might consider:

- Reduce your intake of calories, especially the amount of saturated fat you eat, by substituting lean chicken and fish for red meats and choosing colorful and nutritious vegetables (see Step 5).
- Lose 5 to 7 percent of your body weight—if you weigh around 200 lb now, that's about 10 to 14 lb.
- Increase your physical activity by, for example, walking to the store. An ideal level of exercise is a brisk 30-minute walk, five days each week.

inside information
the polypill

What if a single pill taken daily could slash the incidence of cardiovascular disease? That was the idea of two professors of preventive medicine, Nicholas Wald and Malcolm Law, back in 2003. Their pill would combine a statin with blood pressure-lowering drugs, aspirin and folate to simultaneously reduce four cardiovascular risk factors: "bad" LDL cholesterol, blood pressure, homocysteine and platelet function (which is involved in blood clotting). The idea generated controversy, but now polypill trials have started in six countries. Dubbed the Red Heart pill, it incorporates aspirin, a statin and two blood-pressure drugs. Early results from a trial in India, involving more than 2,000 people, were promising. Maybe the widespread use of a polypill really could, in the original words of Wald and Law, "have a greater impact on the prevention of disease in the Western world than any other single intervention."

TAKING ACTION

The more you understand about atherosclerosis—from the moment when plaque gets deposited in your arteries, to the complex conditions that underlie cardiovascular disease—the better your chances of finding ways to prevent, halt or even reverse it. As already indicated, the damage can frequently be averted by adjusting your lifestyle in relatively small and easy ways that can make a huge difference to your health.

Knowing what you are up against, and accepting that these risks could potentially affect us all, is the first crucial step. In Step 2, we will show you how to recognize an emergency and, just as importantly, explain the most effective action you can take to save your life or the lives of others.

Later on, you will discover a host of ways to assess your own vulnerability to cardiovascular disease, in order to create your own personalized plan of progressive lifestyle changes to lower your risk of heart attacks and strokes. If you make the right lifestyle choices, you may never have to face the threat of either event.

MYTHS X

POTATOES COUNT AS VEGETABLES

No they don't—at least, not in terms of the five to ten portions of fruit and veggies that are recommended as a daily target to protect against cancer, heart disease and strokes. Potatoes may be both delicious and healthy (when not fried), but in nutritional terms they are starchy carbohydrates, more like rice or bread.

But canned or frozen vegetables do count—something that three-quarters of parents didn't know when surveyed. Dried fruits also count and pure fruit juice can count as one portion, but no more than one.

People seem confused—this might be why only about a third of Americans manage to eat five portions of fruit and vegetables per day, according to a survey by the US Centers for Disease Control and Prevention. In Canada, where the target is seven to ten servings, Canadians average 5.16 servings per day. For advice on how to introduce more fruit and vegetables into your diet, see Step 5.

Frozen vegetables do count towards your daily target.

self-defense plan
STEP
2

HOWEVER MUCH YOU KNOW ABOUT RISK FACTORS, AN ACTUAL HEART ATTACK OR STROKE IS A SHOCKING WAKE-UP CALL. IN BOTH CASES, TIME IS OF THE ESSENCE, SO WATCH FOR DANGER SIGNS AND LEARN WHAT YOU CAN DO QUICKLY TO SAVE YOUR OWN LIFE OR THE LIVES OF OTHERS.

Recognize
the danger signs

This step opens with a challenge. You may think you know what happens when someone has a heart attack or stroke – but do you really? Just consider: In the United States, somebody dies from a heart disease-related event every minute, and from a stroke every 3 to 4 minutes. In Canada, the heart disease and stroke rates have fallen 25 percent over the past decade, but together they still claim a life every 7 minutes.

Too often, people think that the only sign of heart attack is pain, but that's not the case at all. If you don't recognize the signs of a heart attack, you may put your own or your loved ones' lives at risk by not taking the correct action. The same is true of strokes; swift treatment can not only save a life, but also prevent long-term disability.

The following pages outline vital information that could help you to control a crisis and make the right decisions in an emergency. You'll learn all about the danger signals, and find out what you could do instantly that might make all the difference. You'll begin to understand why early medical intervention is essential. And you'll discover some of the modern medical miracles—from clot-busting drugs to intricate surgery—that can minimize the damage that a heart attack or stroke may cause.

BLOCKED BLOOD SUPPLY

As explained in Step 1, the underlying causes of most strokes and heart attacks are similar, and the ensuing damage usually results from an interruption of the blood supply to a vital organ. When the blood supply is cut off, cells starved of oxygen and vital nutrients start to die.

If this occurs in the heart, the muscle cells supplied by the blocked artery can no longer function. If the blood supply is not restored quickly, parts of the muscle may die, leaving the heart permanently weakened. Sometimes, the

Strokes are largely preventable, but your risk is a little higher if a grandparent, parent or sibling has had one.

the myths about
heart attacks and strokes

The statements below are common fallacies. Find out why.

- **If you don't have chest pain, you can't be having a heart attack: False.** In a heart attack, blood supply to the heart muscle is interrupted and heart muscle cells start to die, which may cause chest pain—but not necessarily. About one in three people admitted to the hospital with a heart attack does not have severe chest pain.
- **A heart attack gives you sudden, intense pain: Not always.** In some people it does—as in the classic "TV heart attack," where actors clutch their chest in agony. But most real heart attacks build up more slowly, with milder pain or discomfort.
- **If you're worried you may be having a heart attack or stroke, you should call your doctor: False.** Call an ambulance immediately.
- **Heart attacks are rare in women: False.** In fact, a woman is four times more likely to die from a heart attack than from breast cancer; after menopause, heart attacks kill more women than men.
- **Strokes cannot be prevented: False.** Strokes are largely preventable. Quitting smoking, reducing high blood pressure, losing excess weight and getting regular exercise all drastically reduce risk. A landmark 2009 study involving more than 20,000 adults revealed that people who either smoked, drank excessively, were inactive or ate few or no fruits or vegetables were more than twice as likely to suffer a stroke.
- **There's no effective treatment for a stroke: False.** That's why doctors tell you to get to the hospital as soon as possible. For the most common type of stroke, caused by a blood clot, treatment with clot-busting drugs within 4½ hours can significantly reduce the chance of death or permanent disability—the sooner you get them, the better.
- **Strokes only affect old people: False.** On the contrary, more than a quarter of strokes occur in people under the age of 65. Even children can be affected, though this is very rare.
- **Strokes do not run in the family: False.** Your risk of a stroke rises if a parent, grandparent or sibling has had a stroke, especially if they had high blood pressure.
- **Stroke recovery is not possible after the first few weeks: False.** While the most significant improvements occur in the early weeks, recovery can continue for months, even years, particularly if care and rehabilitation begin early.

heart's rhythm becomes irregular, or it may even stop—which, unless someone can get it pumping again, is fatal.

Similarly, if cells in your brain are deprived of their blood supply, they too become damaged. Your brain may no longer be able to issue instructions to other parts of your body. Whatever function is controlled by those damaged brain cells—movement or speech, for example—is suddenly impaired. If blood flow is not rapidly restored and brain cells in one area start to die off, the damage may be permanent.

don't delay

Why do so many people who have heart attacks fail to realize what they are experiencing? One reason is that symptoms can be confusing. A patient may say, "I just didn't feel sick." Some people cannot believe that a heart attack could happen to them, particularly if they are fit and active. So they put off seeking medical help. As many as one in three heart attack patients dies before reaching the hospital—yet these are often lives that might have been saved if the patients, or those around them, had recognized the signs. Immediate action greatly increases your chances of survival. Read on for all possible heart attack and stroke symptoms.

troubleshooting Q&A

I get angina. How could I tell if I was having a heart attack?

Most pain caused by angina is alleviated by rest. So, if you experience chest pain that either starts when you are sitting down or doesn't get better when you stop what you are doing, think heart attack. Similarly, if the pain is more severe than usual, or if it continues for more than 20 minutes or after you've taken your medication, you should call an ambulance. Other symptoms may include nausea and sweating.

TIME AND THE BRAIN

If someone appears to have had a stroke, rapid hospital admission is important so that doctors can run tests to find out how serious the damage is and what caused it. They can then select the right emergency treatment in order to prevent permanent disability.

Sometimes stroke symptoms occur temporarily, disappearing after a few minutes or hours. This is called a TIA (transient ischemic attack, or mini-stroke), and also requires urgent medical attention. A TIA, which is caused by a temporary reduction in the blood supply to part of the brain, is an important warning; without treatment, it is estimated that one in four people who've had a TIA could suffer a full-blown stroke within a month.

Anyone who has experienced a TIA and is deemed to be at high risk of having a full stroke should see a specialist within 24 hours of the onset of symptoms to find out the best course of action.

HELP AT HAND

If you live alone and believe you may be at risk of a heart attack or stroke, consider getting a medical alert system that can be worn around your neck or wrist. These systems communicate with emergency operators who can summon help to your home within minutes.

cardiac crisis

A heart attack may be caused either by ruptured plaque (see page 19) leading to a clot in a coronary artery, or by another event that cuts off vital blood supplies to heart muscle. The medical term for a heart attack is "myocardial infarction," often shortened to MI, which indicates that some cells in the heart muscle (myocardium) have died because of lack of blood (an infarction). In the worst cases, the heart stops beating altogether and goes into cardiac arrest. But, with rapid treatment, damage to the heart muscle can be halted and, if blood flow is restored in time, a full recovery is possible. Otherwise, a part of the heart muscle will be permanently damaged, leaving an area of scar tissue. If the scar tissue is extensive, you may experience long-term breathlessness.

EFFECTIVE TREATMENT

Sometimes a heart attack can disturb the flow of electrical impulses that normally generate your heartbeat and set off the sequence of regular heart muscle contractions that drives blood

REDalert

YOU MAY NOT HAVE CHEST PAIN

People experience heart attacks in different ways. In one major study of 400,000 people over four years, published in the *Journal of the American Medical Association*, one in three patients admitted to the hospital with what was later confirmed to be a heart attack had no chest pain at all. Women and diabetics were among those least likely to have typical symptoms, more than half of whom had no chest pain. According to Dr. Ghada Mikhail, a consulting cardiologist, women are more likely to suffer unusual fatigue, shortness of breath, back pain or abdominal pain.

taking action—heart attacks

It is not always easy to tell whether someone is having a heart attack. But intervention could save the life of someone close to you. It is often up to those around the victim to spot the signs and take urgent action. If you are unsure, don't hesitate. Call 911 and make it clear that it's a suspected heart attack. Ambulance staff would far rather come and tell you it's not, than be called too late.

WHEN SECONDS COUNT

Research has shown that treatment started within an hour of the onset of symptoms reduces the risk of death and lessens damage to the heart. The British Heart Foundation estimates that people who receive medical help within this timeframe are three times more likely to survive a heart attack. That is why it's important to recognize the symptoms, and why, if you suspect that someone is having a heart attack, you should call an ambulance within 5 minutes.

COMMON SYMPTOMS MAY INCLUDE:

- Central chest pain
- Dull, aching discomfort or heaviness in the chest—often mistaken for indigestion
- Pain spreading to the arms, neck or jaw
- Nausea, feeling sick
- Feeling of impending doom
- Sweating, feeling cold and clammy to the touch
- Shortness of breath

LESS COMMON SYMPTOMS MAY INCLUDE:

- A sensation of squeezing or pressure around the chest
- Feeling generally unwell along with chest pain
- Pain in the chest that spreads to the back or abdomen
- Dizziness, feeling faint or light-headed, along with chest pain
- In women: pain in the back, jaw or abdomen, or unusual fatigue

SYMPTOMS CAN DECEIVE

Symptoms of a heart attack vary from one person to another and may be less obvious in women than in men. Diabetics are more likely to have a "silent" attack, without chest pain; instead they may suffer shortness of breath, nausea, faintness or loss of consciousness.

early morning alarm

You might think that heart attacks and strokes would tend to strike when you're tired at the end of the day. In fact, both occur most frequently in the early hours of daylight. Heart attacks are 40 percent more common between 6 a.m. and noon than at other times of day, and more than 45 percent of strokes occur during these hours. Similarly, sudden cardiac deaths are 29 percent more common in the morning, and serious rhythm disturbances, heart failure deaths and ruptured aortic aneurysms follow a similar pattern.

There are numerous reasons why the first few hours after waking are so hazardous. Stress hormones such as adrenaline and cortisol, as well as the male hormone testosterone, peak in the early morning in preparation for the day and cause an increase in heart rate and blood pressure. Relative dehydration overnight and an increase in platelet "stickiness" make blood clots more likely, and the effects of medication taken at bedtime may be wearing off.

So it makes sense to get up gradually and allow time for a leisurely start to the day. Have a long, relaxing stretch and preferably a warm-up before you start moving about. Avoid sudden bouts of exertion first thing, especially if you are not particularly fit, and especially in very cold weather (another trigger for heart attacks and strokes).

Stretch and get up slowly in the morning.

It's also important to stay as calm as possible and not to get upset about problems at work or the frustrations of commuting. Study the destressing techniques in Step 9. Check with your doctor that any medications you take will last the night, and make sure to time your last doses of the day accordingly.

troubleshooting Q&A

I have high blood pressure and I like to run in the morning. Am I increasing my risk of a heart attack?

No, not if you are used to exercising regularly. It is only sudden, infrequent exertion that poses the greatest hazard to health. And that fact appears to hold true even if you already have heart disease. According to a study of patients who had had a heart attack and later took part in a cardiac rehabilitation program, there was no significant difference in the rate of complications whether the patients exercised at 7:30 in the morning or 3 o'clock in the afternoon. The patients always followed a stretching and warm-up routine before doing exercise, with a cool-down period afterwards—following a golden rule for anyone who exercises (see Step 7).

around your body. If this happens, you may develop heart-rhythm abnormalities, known as arrhythmias.

Arrhythmias are most common in the first three to six hours following an attack. Some are mild, but they may cause palpitations, dizziness, chest pain, shortness of breath or fatigue. Others can be life-threatening. If you are in the hospital, arrhythmias can be detected and treated—another reason for seeking prompt emergency assistance.

If damage to the heart muscle is extensive, heart failure may follow. Your heart cannot pump strongly enough to propel blood around your body, and you are likely to experience breathlessness that may become severe as fluid accumulates in your lungs.

Heart failure can usually be diagnosed quickly from the symptoms, a physical examination and various tests. It can also be treated effectively in the hospital with drugs that lower blood pressure, prevent further heart muscle damage and reduce the heart's workload. However, severe cases may need surgery to bypass the blocked coronary artery and restore blood flow.

ASPIRIN

Chewing one 325 mg standard aspirin tablet in those crucial moments before an ambulance arrives can help to minimize the damage caused by a heart attack.

Aspirin works by reducing the "stickiness" of the platelets that are an important part of the body's blood-clotting mechanism, and so may stop a dangerous clot from progressing. But aspirin should not be taken for a suspected stroke in case it is hemorrhagic (caused by bleeding), which aspirin could exacerbate.

- Don't take aspirin if you are allergic to it, or if you are taking warfarin or other anti-clotting drugs.
- If you are with someone who is having a heart attack, check that the person is not allergic to aspirin, then ask where you can find some.
- If you are on your own, take aspirin only if there is some nearby. Do not search the house—you need to stay still.
- Take one aspirin tablet and chew it slowly instead of swallowing it. This is a faster way to get the drug into your bloodstream.

Aspirin works by reducing the "stickiness" of the platelets that are an important part of the body's blood-clotting mechanism

Don't hesitate to call emergency services if you or anyone around you may be experiencing a heart attack or stroke.

what happens during a stroke?

There are two main types of strokes and each requires very different treatment, so doctors have to pinpoint the type as soon as possible. The first and most common type is an ischemic stroke, which is like a heart attack: a blood clot blocks one of the arteries supplying the brain, cutting the blood supply to brain cells that control functions such as speech or movement. The other type, known as a hemorrhagic stroke, occurs when an artery wall leaks, causing bleeding in the brain. In both cases, the results are similar: The patient's brain cells are unable to perform their usual control functions and could die, leading to permanent disability, unless intervention is swift.

INSIDE YOUR BRAIN

Changes to the connections between brain cells begin to occur within 3 minutes of the onset of stroke symptoms, according to animal research carried out by Canadian scientists. But, with prompt treatment to restore blood flow, 94 percent of these connections can be repaired.

That is why it is so crucial for a stroke victim to get to the hospital quickly. The sooner you are assessed and treated, the better your chances of a full recovery.

taking action—strokes

If you think that you or someone near you may be having a stroke, call 911. Ask for an ambulance and make it clear to the emergency operator that the person may have suffered from a stroke. More importantly, tell the paramedics when the ambulance arrives. They will then take you to the nearest hospital with a stroke unit, avoiding life-threatening delays.

ACT FAST

The effects of a stroke can be felt in almost any part of the body. Yet someone who has just suffered one will probably be extremely confused and not realize what is happening or be able to act quickly. It is often up to family, friends or caretakers to recognize a stroke and get help fast.

NO WARNING

Symptoms of a stroke come on suddenly. Since people who are experiencing a stroke frequently rely on those around them to spot what's happening, the American Stroke Association and the Heart and Stroke Foundation of Canada both urge everyone to know the five warning signs of strokes:

Sudden weakness, numbness or paralysis on one side of the face, one arm or one leg, even if it's only temporary.

Sudden difficulty speaking or understanding, or general confusion, even if it's only temporary.

Sudden trouble seeing, even if it's only temporary.

Sudden severe headache.

Sudden dizziness or loss of balance.

If someone close to you experiences any of these symptoms, call 911 immediately.

Owain Wyn-Jones

A fast response

Owain Wyn-Jones will be for ever grateful that someone very close to him knew how to recognize a stroke. Because Laraine Adams - then his girlfriend, now his wife - spotted the telltale signs of a stroke, he reached the hospital in 40 minutes, well within the $4\frac{1}{2}$ hours during which clot-busting treatment is most effective.

"We'd been at our friends' house for dinner the night before," says Laraine, "and we drank a lot of wine. When Owain got up the next day, he said he felt like he was still drunk. He stumbled a bit and had a headache. As we sat having a cup of coffee, he leaned over and put his head on my shoulder. When he sat up, I noticed his face had fallen on one side."

Luckily, they'd seen a public service announcement about the warning signs of strokes. "I remembered it because we thought it was so shocking." She asked Owain to lift up both arms. "He couldn't lift his left one. And he couldn't stand up, because his left leg gave way under him when he tried. I thought it was a stroke, but it was hard to believe," she said, particularly since Owain was just 30 years old. Still, she called 911, and was told to get Owain to the closest stroke unit, a hospital

'There is a very short window in which a stroke can be treated, so acting quickly is imperative.'

about 10 minutes from their home.

The ambulance took Owain to a nearby hospital. There, doctors treated him with a clot-busting drug to dissolve the blood clot causing his symptoms. He stayed in the hospital another four days for observation and some rehabilitation.

Owain had no apparent risk factors, but stress, says Laraine, may have played a part. "He was worried about his business and was working very long hours."

Since then he has been forced to take things much easier. He still has problems with memory and concentration. The couple feel strongly that everyone should be aware of stroke symptoms.

"If you suspect it, don't feel you may be wasting doctors' time," urges Laraine. "There is a very short window in which a stroke can be treated, so acting quickly is imperative."

while you wait for help

Remind yourself that most people survive a heart attack or stroke. Once you have called 911, you can improve the odds of recovery by knowing exactly what to do before the paramedics arrive. Crucially, the patient must stay still and calm to minimize the pressure on the cardiovascular system and reduce the amount of oxygen the body requires.

IF YOU ARE ALONE

- Unlock the front door so it can be opened from outside.
- Stay calm.
- Sit or lie down.
- Have the phone ready, next to you.
- Do not eat or drink anything other than small sips of water.
- Call a neighbor or family member to wait with you if possible.

WHAT YOU CAN DO TO HELP

- Don't leave the person alone.
- Help him or her to sit or lie down to be more comfortable.
- Check the time; this information may be helpful to the ambulance crew.
- Offer reassurance that the ambulance is on its way.
- Don't give food or drinks, besides water (except when the patient has medication to take in case of an attack—in which case, give it at once).
- Call the person's doctor; information about past medical history may be helpful to the ambulance crew and hospital doctors.
- If possible, gather all the patient's current medication so that this can be sent to the hospital with the patient.
- If you know about basic first aid, do an ABC check: Airways, Breathing and Circulation.
- If the patient vomits, turn the head to one side to reduce choking risk.
- Watch out for signs of cardiac arrest, where the heart stops beating altogether. The person will stop breathing and will not have a pulse. Be prepared to start resuscitation.
- If the person is unconscious, place in the recovery position (see page 48), but continue to watch breathing to see if resuscitation is needed.

SECRETweapon

A STROKE UNIT

If you suspect that you or someone close to you may be having a stroke or mini-stroke, it is important to try to get to a hospital with a certified stroke unit. Such units include a multi-disciplinary team of doctors, nurses and therapists skilled in the field of stroke medicine, which can greatly improve recovery prospects.

Just like heart attacks, strokes must be treated as medical emergencies. A stroke unit can provide rapid and early diagnosis, vital to saving lives. If tests show that your stroke is due to a blood clot, a drug given within 4½ hours of the onset of symptoms greatly improves your chance of a full recovery, and the earlier it is given, the better.

recovery position

If someone is unconscious but breathing, he or she should be put into the recovery position to keep the airway open and ensure there is no risk of choking. If the victim is lying flat, bend the arm nearest to you upwards, so the forearm is at right angles to the upper arm, then lay the other arm across the chest. Support the head and gently roll the person towards you onto his or her side, with the head resting on the arm that was across the chest. Bend the upper leg to prevent the victim from rolling too far. Check the pulse and breathing regularly until medical help arrives.

life-saving skills

If someone collapses with a heart attack or cardiac arrest, their chances of survival more than double if a bystander performs cardiopulmonary resuscitation (CPR) to keep the heart beating. If the heart stops during an attack, the patient may lose consciousness and will die within minutes if blood flow to the brain and other vital organs is not restored. CPR buys time. When the ambulance arrives, paramedics may be able to restart the heart with an electric shock, a process known as defibrillation.

Conventional CPR involves two elements: chest compressions to keep blood pumping through the heart, combined with mouth-to-mouth breathing to maintain a flow of air into the lungs. However, compression-only CPR is rapidly gaining favor—especially for those untrained in CPR.

MAKING IT EASIER TO HELP

Fewer than one in three people who have a heart attack in public is helped by a bystander. Why is this? Well, some people don't know what to do, while others may be put off by the mouth-to-mouth element. New guidelines by the American Heart Association and the Heart and Stroke Foundation of Canada have changed the ABCs (Airway, Breathing, Chest compressions) to a newer system that starts with the chest compression. For untrained bystanders, the new guidelines call for compression only.

compression-only CPR

1 Kneel beside the victim and, if necessary, roll him or her onto the back. Find the lower end of the ribcage and run your first two fingers inwards until you find the bottom of the breastbone. Place your index finger at this point as a marker. Place the heel of your other hand on the breastbone just above this finger and maintain this position.

Push down vertically with your arms straight.

2 Move your other hand on top of the first and interlace the fingers of both hands. Lean forwards, with your shoulders over the patient. Keeping your arms straight, push down, aiming to press the lower breastbone down by at least two inches, and continue at a compression rate of at least 100 compressions per minute. Release the pressure without removing your hands. If you are unwilling or unable to give mouth-to-mouth ventilation, continue with compression-only CPR until EMS specialists take over.

the Bee Gees

Don't know how fast to perform chest compressions? Make sure that you're familiar with the 1977 Bee Gees hit "Staying Alive." It has 103 beats per minute, close enough to the 100-per-minute ideal rhythm for chest compressions in cardiopulmonary resuscitation (CPR). Researchers played the song to 15 doctors and medical students learning CPR on dummies, and told them to time their chest compressions to the beat. Five weeks later they were tested without the music, but asked simply to recall the "Staying Alive" rhythm while performing compressions. They achieved impressive average compression rates of 109 to 113 beats per minute. Many people hesitate to undertake CPR because they're not sure of the rhythm, but performing CPR properly can triple the survival rate after a heart attack—so "Staying Alive" could help someone to do just that.

When doctors in Tokyo studied 4,068 people who were not in the hospital when they suffered cardiac arrest, they noted the number who had received CPR from bystanders, including compression-only CPR. After assessing the degree of brain damage among survivors 30 days later, they reported that more than twice as many had "a favorable neurological outcome" when resuscitation had been attempted.

UNEXPECTED RESULTS

What really surprised them was that among those who had stopped breathing and for whom resuscitation had begun within 4 minutes of their heart attack, compression-only resuscitation produced a better outcome than full CPR, more than doubling the number who survived without brain damage. Adding mouth-to-mouth respiration showed no benefit in any of the patient groups studied.

The American Heart Association and the Heart and Stroke Foundation of Canada agree that, for people untrained in CPR, it may be preferable to do chest compressions only.

DEFENSEtactics

TRAINING

Resuscitation is easy—if you know how to do it. So why not find out? Both the Canadian Red Cross and American Red Cross offer CPR training and certification in communities throughout their respective countries. To find a class near you, or to schedule a class for several people, go to redcross.org or redcross.ca. Once trained, CPR certificates are valid for one year.

Keith Lawrenz

Saving a life

When Keith Lawrenz, 43, collapsed in the street, he had good fortune on his side. Peter Marchant, a first aid volunteer who is fully trained in CPR, worked nearby.

"I was at work and someone came running in and told me that a man had collapsed round the corner," Peter recalls. "I noticed that his lips were blue and he was gasping with agonal breathing." (Irregular or "agonal" gasps can occur during cardiac arrest.)

Keith's heart had stopped, so Peter immediately rolled him onto his back and began CPR. While he performed chest compressions, he called out to one of the bystanders to give mouth-to-mouth, and another to check that an ambulance was on its way. When the ambulance arrived 5 minutes later, Peter was asked to continue the compressions while the paramedics tried to restart Keith's heart with a defibrillator and drugs. A second ambulance crew arrived and took over CPR while the first crew repeated their attempts. After the second shock, Keith's heart restarted.

He was then rushed to the hospital and Peter didn't expect to hear any more about it. But the next day, he was told that

"I noticed that his lips were blue and he was gasping with agonal breathing." Keith's heart had stopped.

Keith and his wife were trying to contact him.

When Peter went to see him in the hospital, Keith thanked him warmly and said, "Everyone keeps calling me the miracle around here, but you're a part of that."

Peter was given an award in recognition of his dramatic intervention. Keith's heart had stopped for 24 minutes. He went on to make a full recovery, where without Peter's efforts he would likely have died.

"I was absolutely elated to find out that he was OK," Peter says. "My training ensured that I was able to keep him alive."

YOUR BLOOD

When diagnosing a possible heart attack in a patient who may have symptoms such as chest pains, medical staff are aware that speed is of the essence. First they will take an ECG (electrocardiogram, also called an EKG) to record the heart's electrical impulses and to detect an irregular rhythm or other abnormalities that indicate a heart attack. But if the ECG is inconclusive, blood tests are performed which will reveal if the heart muscle has sustained any damage. Such blood tests are usually taken within two to three hours, and then repeated up to 12 hours after a suspected attack.

What they measure is the level of an enzyme called troponin, which is released into the bloodstream if the heart muscle is damaged or dying. The second blood test is routine to confirm the results. If the tests are positive, doctors will determine the best treatment. If negative, the patient is usually sent home.

how hospitals save lives

When treating a heart attack or stroke, doctors have three urgent aims: to save a life, ease pain, and keep the heart muscle or brain from permanent harm. If an ambulance has been called, the attending crew will assess the patient en route to the hospital and feed doctors back as much information as they can so that treatment can begin immediately.

heart treatment

If you are rushed to the hospital with a suspected heart attack, the first actions of the medical staff will be to attach you to a cardiac monitor and an intravenous drip. You will then be given oxygen and pain-relief medication while an electrocardiogram (ECG) test is performed to trace the electrical activity of your heart. Staff will also take a sample of your blood, which will be tested for the presence of enzymes released from

life-saving heart surgery

ANGIOPLASTY

If you reach the hospital quickly, doctors may try to open up your coronary arteries mechanically. This is known as percutaneous intervention (PCI) or angioplasty, and is the preferred option if time permits. A thin tube with a balloon at the tip is threaded up from your groin or wrist and into your coronary artery. A small amount of dye is injected so that the site of the blockage can be seen using an X-ray video (a test called a coronary angiogram) and the balloon is inflated to widen the artery. The tube is then withdrawn, although a small metal coil known as a stent is usually left in place in the artery to keep it open and prevent further blockages. Some stents even release drugs to help keep the artery clear.

BYPASS SURGERY

Angioplasty is successful in opening up about 90 percent of clogged arteries. It rapidly relieves pain and can reduce damage to the heart muscle. However, for some conditions, this procedure is not suitable. If your main coronary artery is blocked, or if you have multiple blockages or a complicating condition such as diabetes, doctors may decide to perform an immediate coronary artery bypass graft (CABG) instead.

A CABG entails open-heart surgery, a major procedure. A healthy blood vessel taken from elsewhere in the body is linked to the two ends of your coronary artery on either side of a blockage, to provide an alternative passage for blood to flow to your heart muscle. Often, two or three coronary arteries are bypassed during the same operation.

damaged heart muscle. And all this will take place within minutes of your arrival in the emergency room. Doctors may start treatment while waiting for the results of the blood tests. You may be given aspirin or put on a heparin drip—both have blood-thinning, anti-clotting properties.

If doctors suspect that your symptoms are due to a spasm of a coronary artery (see page 19), they may inject a drug to try to relieve this. If your heart rhythm is abnormal, you may be given medication or electric shocks, or a temporary pacemaker may be implanted under your skin to control your heartbeat.

HEALING DRUGS

Doctors may also give you thrombolytic drugs like streptokinase or reteplase to dissolve the clot blocking the coronary artery and restore blood flow to the heart.

Thrombolytic drugs work by attacking fibrin, the substance in your blood that keeps a clot together. The sooner the drugs are given, the more likely they are to prevent permanent damage to your heart muscle. They are most effective when administered within the first three to four hours (preferably within the first hour) following the onset of symptoms. However, they will give satisfactory results up to six hours after and still have some benefit up to 12 hours after symptoms have first appeared.

SPECIAL DELIVERY

Thrombolytic or clot-busting drugs have revolutionised the treatment of heart attacks. These drugs are effective in opening up the coronary arteries in about half of all patients, reducing damage and improving the chances of long-term survival.

In some areas, ambulance paramedics responding to suspected heart-attack calls now carry thrombolytic drugs with them, so that they can be administered straight away (after an ECG test has been carried out, to confirm the heart attack). When the patient arrives in the hospital, doctors will monitor his or her condition carefully, since clot-busting drugs can promote bleeding.

stroke treatment

If you have a stroke, the emergency services will usually take you to the nearest hospital with a specialist stroke unit or a specialised stroke team, because immediate expert assessment and treatment is important to ensure the best possible outcome.

On arrival, you would have your blood pressure measured and an ECG to check for abnormal heart rhythms. Blood samples are taken to test for diabetes, high cholesterol or blood clotting problems and other conditions.

The doctors' first priority is to identify the type of stroke: whether it was triggered by a clot or bleeding. If the stroke was triggered by bleeding, it would be extremely dangerous to administer an anti-clotting drug.

...immediate expert assessment and treatment is important to ensure the best possible outcome.

One or more of the following diagnostic tests may be used to identify the type of stroke: either ischemic (caused by a blood clot) or hemorrhagic (caused by bleeding):

- Computed tomography (CT) scan—a scan based on multiple X-rays, which is used to produce a 3D picture that can confirm the diagnosis of a stroke and demonstrate whether it was caused by bleeding in the brain.
- Magnetic resonance imaging (MRI) scan—a scan that creates pictures generated by a magnetic field, used to identify the precise location of the stroke and help medical staff to decide on further therapy.
- Cerebral angiogram—a special X-ray taken after the injection of a dye into the arteries supplying the brain. It provides a detailed map of the blood flow to the brain, revealing where there is a blockage or bleeding within the brain's blood supply.

RESUPPLYING THE BRAIN

If a stroke is found to have been caused by a blood clot, you may be given a thrombolytic drug to dissolve the clot, assuming you receive it within 4½ hours of the start of your symptoms. Any longer and the risk of bleeding outweighs the benefits of dissolving the clot. You'll likely be given antithrombotic drugs like aspirin, dipyridamole (Persantine) or clopidogrel (Plavix). Up to 6 hours after a stroke, a clot-busting drug can be delivered via a catheter directly to the site of the blockage, or the clot can be removed with a device thet extracts, dissolves or breaks it up.

If, after a non-disabling ischemic stroke or a TIA, tests identify a substantial blockage in the carotid artery, doctors may suggest an operation to open up the artery in order to reduce the risk of another stroke. You may also need medication to reduce blood pressure and blood clotting, and to lower cholesterol.

TREATING BLEEDING

In patients who reach the hospital after a hemorrhagic stroke, the original bleeding has usually stopped. To reduce the risk of further bleeding, doctors monitor blood pressure carefully and prescribe medication to keep it under control. If doctors think that your stroke is related to taking aspirin or an anticoagulant like warfarin, you may be given a drug to reverse its effects. Occasionally in the case of bleeding, surgery may be suggested to drain the blood from your brain, though this isn't suitable for everyone. Open surgery or keyhole surgery may also be advised to seal a cerebral aneurysm if this is what has caused the bleeding.

Recovery can continue for months, even years. The brain is a remarkable organ. Some studies have shown improvements up to 14 years later.

the road to recovery

When the patient's condition has been stabilized, the process of recovery begins. For most people, it takes time to adjust. Your heart may be going through changes as part of the healing process, and doctors will want to monitor you closely to make sure that you do not develop signs of heart failure or heart rhythm abnormalities. You may be referred for tests to assess if further treatment could reduce your risk of another attack.

BRAIN REPAIR

Some recovery from the physical symptoms of strokes may happen while you are still in the hospital, but it is a process that can continue for months, even years. The brain is a remarkable organ. After a stroke, recovery occurs partly as a result of brain cells which were temporarily damaged starting to function again, and partly as a result of other parts of the brain unaffected by the stroke taking over the functions of the damaged area. Some studies have shown improvements in neural function up to 14 years later. During the recovery period, you'll receive help from a range of key health professionals, both in the hospital and at home, whose input will be crucial to your successful rehabilitation.

GOING HOME

When you're discharged from the hospital, you will be prescribed medication that you will probably have to take for the foreseeable future to protect against further attacks. Both heart and stroke patients may require blood pressure-lowering drugs, aspirin and other anti-platelet drugs that prevent blood clots from occurring in the future, as well as cholesterol-lowering drugs. Others may also require drugs for conditions such as diabetes and abnormal heart rhythms.

It is important to follow your doctors' instructions and take all medications exactly as prescribed.

READY FOR REHAB

People who have had a heart attack or stroke begin a rehabilitation program as soon as possible. In the case of strokes, the program may begin 24 to 48 hours after the stroke, while you're still hospitalized. The program will likely include some excersise, healthy-living advice and general tips on how to maintain a healthy heart. See **cardiachealth.ca** or **heartandstroke.com** for more information.

The length of rehab varies depending on your individual situation. In the case of a severely disabling stroke, it may last years.

Research indicates that a cardiac rehabilitation program after a heart attack can improve five-year survival rates by about 26 percent. Therapists can help people to make adjustments to their lifestyle—such as

SECRETweapon

OPTIMISM

There is powerful evidence to suggest that, if your general outlook is optimistic, you have a lower risk of heart attacks, strokes and death from cardiovascular disease than someone who is constantly negative about life. And if you have already had a heart attack and yet remain positive about the future, you are three times less likely to suffer a second attack than those with a more pessimistic response.

In one study that followed the fortunes of 122 men who had had a heart attack, 21 of the 25 dyed-in-the-wool pessimists had died eight years after the attack, compared with just six out of 25 confirmed optimists.

Another study of 309 patients who had undergone coronary artery bypass graft surgery showed that optimistic patients were only half as likely as pessimistic ones to be rehospitalised with complications including infection, angina, a repeat heart attack or the need for more surgery.

SEE YOUR DOCTOR

Enlist the help of your doctor in your fight back against cardiovascular disease. Your doctor is in charge of your overall medical care when you come out of the hospital, and it's important to see him or her for regular follow-ups. Tell your doctor if you're experiencing any new symptoms or having problems with side effects of medication.

Think of your local doctor as a vital resource. Your doctor can help you to find a local rehabilitation program that suits you (some centers ask for a doctor referral). He or she can tell you about fitness plans run by local hospitals or medical centers. Depending on your needs, your doctor can also put you in touch with community health services or social services, and can arrange for a community or district nurse to make regular visits. (See Resources, page 240.)

giving up smoking, adopting a healthier diet, losing weight and getting fit—and can also help patients deal with the anxiety and depression that are common after a heart attack.

Rehabilitation is crucial for stroke patients, too. Many people make a full recovery, but others have some lasting impairment and may need help with day-to-day living. A rehabilitation team may include physiotherapists, speech therapists and occupational therapists who help people to regain function or cope with problems that can affect walking, talking, dressing or writing.

FIGHTING BACK TO FITNESS

An essential part of rehabilitation is to help you to reduce your risk of having a heart attack or a stroke in the future. Remaining positive is part of that process. So remember:

- If you survive a heart attack, there is an 18 percent chance that you could have a second one within three years—or, if you look at it another way, a 72 percent chance that you won't.
- Similarly, if you survive a stroke, you have a 25 percent chance of suffering another within 5 years, or a 75 percent chance that you won't.

There are countless ways in which lifestyle changes can cut your cardiovascular risk. Here are a few things to consider:

- Having a stressful job more than doubles your risk of another heart attack within two years of the first one.
- Quitting smoking after a heart attack reduces your risk of a further attack by 32 percent.
- Controlling high blood pressure is especially important, as high blood pressure is a significant risk factor for strokes.
- Increasing your level of physical activity after a heart attack reduces your risk of having another one by 78 percent.

- Moderate exercise and eating five portions of fruit and vegetables a day can reduce stroke risk in men and women by about a quarter.
- Men and women who have one or two glasses of red or white wine per day more than halve their risk of a second heart attack compared with teetotalers. But there is no benefit in exceeding the recommended limits: 1 serving per day for women and 1 to 2 for men. Excess alcohol intake is a well-established risk factor for both heart attack and stroke.

A moderate consumption of wine may halve your risk of a second heart attack— friends help, too …

SECRET weapon

A FRIENDLY CHAT

Don't forget to involve your friends and family in your rehabilitation. Their emotional support can be invaluable at a time when you may be feeling anxious or depressed. There is evidence that it may also lower your risk of having another attack. A study of 600 patients at Manchester Royal Infirmary in England found that people who confided in a close friend, partner or relative after a heart attack halved their risk of another attack during the following 12 months, compared to those without such a strong bond.

Consider joining a support group made up of people who have had heart attacks or strokes. Set up by patients for patients, these groups also give families the chance to meet and talk to people who have been through the same experience as them. Groups meet socially, arrange to take weekend walks together and learn to enjoy life again during the period of recuperation. Check with hospitals or clinics in your area to find one close to you.

GETTING ACTIVE

Doing exercise after you have had a heart attack or a stroke is one of the most important factors in your recovery. But the prospect can seem daunting. Remember that exercise will be recommended only if your doctors judge that you are sufficiently fit.

Before starting an exercise program, heart patients are sometimes asked to undergo an echocardiogram (a test that allows medical staff to visualize the heart by bouncing sound waves off it) to assess their heart function, and a treadmill test to check that that their heart can cope with a moderate exercise routine without problems.

Doctors advocate regular exercise as the best way to strengthen your heart after an attack. Two types in particular are recommended: aerobic exercise—such as walking, jogging, cycling or swimming—and careful resistance (strength) training.

LOOKING TO THE LONG TERM

As discussed in Step 1, atherosclerosis is a disease affecting the whole body. Treating the immediate effects of a heart attack or stroke will not get rid of atherosclerosis, and long-term medication can control the problems it causes only to a limited

The vital thing is to keep active and do regular exercise, so your heart gets used to a gentle workout.

If I've experienced a heart attack, should I avoid having sex?

After you have been given the all-clear to engage in moderate exercise—which your doctors will probably recommend anyway—then having sex is as safe as, say, running up the stairs: Both activities will increase your heart rate to around 130 beats per minute (your heart rate at rest is around 70 beats per minute). Fewer than 1 percent of heart attacks are caused by intercourse, and the risk is no greater for someone with a history of heart attacks or angina than for anyone else.

Most people are able to start having sex again within two to three weeks of having a heart attack. But check with your doctor first if you are still getting chest pains or if you have very high blood pressure or heart rhythm disturbances (which may be signalled by palpitations). Physically fit people are able to enjoy sex with no increased risk.

The vital thing is to keep active and to take regular exercise, so your heart gets used to a gentle workout. The more you exercise, the safer sex becomes.

extent. That is why most people who have had heart attacks are advised by their doctors to make alterations to their lifestyle that will reduce the risk of further attacks.

Many of the lifestyle changes that doctors suggest for people at risk of or recovering from a heart attack or stroke reflect the advice outlined in this book: Stop smoking, eat healthily, increase your activity levels, lose weight if necessary and avoid stress. You will learn more about all these things in the next chapters.

So, even if you have already had a heart attack or stroke, or if you have been given a timely warning in the form of worsening angina or a mini-stroke, absorbing the advice provided in the following steps will help to boost your recovery and lessen your future risk.

YOUR UNIQUE SURVIVAL KIT

You know how to recognize the vital symptoms of heart disease and strokes and how you can take action to protect yourself and those close to you. Even more importantly, you have learned that swift action makes a difference and can save lives.

Now that you understand the risks, it is time to consider how to make the changes that will give you lifelong protection against cardiovascular disease. Step 3 will give you the tools to examine your current lifestyle in detail, with the aim of identifying ways in which you may be damaging your own health. You can then work out your own risk profile and start to make a range of small adjustments that could have a major and positive impact on your health in the years to come.

self-defense plan

STEP

3

MOST OF US COULD DO SOME SIMPLE THINGS TO IMPROVE THE HEALTH OF OUR HEART AND ARTERIES. NOW IS THE TIME TO FIND OUT IF THE WAY YOU LIVE IS AFFECTING YOUR RISK OF FUTURE PROBLEMS AND IDENTIFY KEY AREAS WHERE SMALL CHANGES CAN MAKE ALL THE DIFFERENCE.

Assess
your risk

The following pages present a series of questionnaires that will help you to assess what effect your lifestyle choices may be having on your health. Once you understand your risk profile, you'll be in a better position to decide which elements of your daily life may need to be modified to give you the best protection against heart disease and strokes.

HOW DOCTORS CALCULATE RISK

As preventive medicine gains ever more prominence in health services, doctors are taking a more proactive role in patient care. For example, if you are over 40, your doctor may invite you to have a "heart health check" to determine your risk of developing cardiovascular disease in the future.

The scoring system doctors generally employ to assess a patient's risk takes account of age, gender, family history, systolic blood pressure (the higher figure, see page 26), blood cholesterol levels and whether he or she smokes. As far as cholesterol is concerned, what matters is the ratio between the total cholesterol and "good" HDL cholesterol (see page 18); the higher the proportion of HDL, the better. A computer program is used to analyze the data that has been collected and to estimate the likelihood of a patient experiencing a heart attack or stroke within the next ten years.

THE BIG PICTURE

When deciding whether to advise drug treatment or make a referral to a cardiologist, a doctor will also note whether the patient already has signs of cardiovascular disease—especially angina—or peripheral arterial disease, or a family history of heart attacks or strokes.

The doctor will look at linked problems such as diabetes or obesity and measure a patient's weight and height. The result gained from these measurements is called body mass index, or BMI. (If you would like to calculate your own BMI, follow the method described on page 66.) The formula that doctors use to estimate risk is complicated, but there are online calculators where you can feed in your own figures and work out your risk (for example, qrisk.org). You will need to know your blood pressure and cholesterol levels (both total cholesterol and HDL cholesterol) but, as both are important health indicators, it is worth asking your doctor to check them, especially if you are over the age of 40.

CAUGHT IN THE WEB

Risk factors tend to be interlinked and can exacerbate each other, so the more risk factors you have, the higher your overall level of risk. In fact, cardiovascular risk resembles an intricate spider's web: Obesity, high blood pressure and diabetes all increase your risk. Obesity combined with a high intake of salt or excessive alcohol consumption also raises the risk of high blood pressure. A poor diet can contribute to obesity, diabetes, high blood pressure and high cholesterol —all of which feed into your overall risk, as well. Stress increases risk both directly and by increasing blood pressure. The older a person is, the more susceptible he or she is to high blood pressure caused by stress at work. And so on.

Habits play a role too, especially smoking,

... smoking increases your risk dramatically

which is specifically highlighted in the risk-prediction charts used by medical staff.

● If you are a man under 50 who is also a non-smoker with normal blood pressure and cholesterol levels, your chance of getting cardiovascular disease within the next ten years is low (less than 10 percent). Change just one element—add a smoking habit, for example—and your risk of heart attacks or strokes rises to between 10 and 20 percent.

● If you are a woman aged between 50 and 59, smoking increases your risk dramatically—pushing it as high as 30 percent if you also have high blood pressure and a high level of "bad" LDL cholesterol in your blood (see page 18).

I'm 67, fit and active, and I eat healthily. Am I still at risk?

Many older people who have a healthy lifestyle remain free of cardiovascular disease—particularly those who are not exposed to the bad diet, sedentary occupations and high levels of stress typical of Western societies. But generally, the risk of developing cardiovascular disease does increase with age, since over the years we reap the consequences of more and more exposure to various factors detrimental to health such as environmental pollution. So the older you are, the more you need to take account of any personal added risk factors that you uncover as you work through this chapter.

DEALING WITH THE HAZARDS OF MODERN LIFE

Nobody can protect themselves against all risks, but there are steps we can take to avoid obvious hazards. For example, minimizing junk food consumption and eating plenty of fruit and vegetables will have a beneficial effect on your blood cholesterol levels and help regulate your blood pressure.

What you eat and drink plays a huge role in your well-being and, in Steps 5 and 6, you'll discover more about the simple dietary rules that make all the difference—replacing animal fats with healthier oils whenever possible, for instance, and keeping your calorie intake under control.

Walking in the country or even your local park will improve your fitness and benefit your heart and lungs. (Air pollution is another enemy of cardiovascular health, as are stressful, excessive noise and the sleep disturbances that comes from both noise and light pollution.) See Step 8 for ten everyday hazards—including plastics that have been linked to cardiovascular disease—and discover how to combat or avoid them.

HEALTHY BALANCE

Reducing stress at work and ensuring that, however deskbound you are, you incorporate activity into your day will also boost your chances of avoiding heart attacks and strokes. In Step 7, you'll discover fitness routines and "deskercises" to counteract the potential harm that a sedentary day can wreak on your body. In Step 9, you'll find out the best ways to tackle stress and learn sleep-promoting strategies and general tactics to enhance your sense of well-being even under pressure.

The goal is to achieve a healthy balance. By knowing that for most activities there is a risk-to-benefit ratio, you can decide which are acceptable, which are avoidable and which you can compensate for.

estimating your risk

The information and questionnaires on the following pages are designed to help you to assess how well you are protecting your heart and arteries in various aspects of your life.

As you work through the sets of questions, you may find it helpful to use a notebook or diary to jot down your scores and your risk assessment, so you can look back and monitor your progress in the coming months as you gradually reduce your risk in different areas. Be honest when you answer, and read on. Step 4 supplies solutions to any problem areas.

your vital statistics

WHAT'S YOUR BMI?

Numerous medical studies confirm that being overweight and carrying too much fat—especially abdominal fat—increases the risk of having a heart attack or stroke. One of the best ways of discovering whether you are overweight is to work out your body mass index, or BMI, a standard formula for measuring body fat (see below). It is a much better measure than weight alone because it takes account of height.

how lean are you?

Calculating your body mass index (BMI) is the best way to assess whether you are overweight for your height. Follow this formula:

CALCULATE YOUR BMI

1 Note your weight in pounds _____, then multiply by 703 = _____

2 Note your height in inches, then square it: _____ x _____ = _____

3 Divide line 1 by line 2: _____ ÷ _____ = **body mass index** _____

A BMI of between 18.5 and 25 is considered healthy. If your BMI is in the 26–30 range, you are classed as overweight. If your BMI is in the 31–40 range, you are obese; if 41 or over, you are severely obese. Note: Muscle weighs more than fat, so people who are very muscular will have a high BMI without the associated health risks.

WATCH YOUR WAIST

Your waist size is also key because it reveals how much fat you have around your abdomen. Find a tape measure and write down your waist circumference. For women, waist size should not exceed 35 in (88 cm); for men, 40 in (101 cm) is the max. These figures should be slightly lower for people of South Asian, Chinese, Japanese, African and South American descent, who have a higher risk of cardiovascular disease.

Even if your BMI is within the healthy range, you may still be at higher risk of developing long-term problems if you carry too much weight in your abdominal area. To find out if you fall into this category, you can calculate your waist-to-hip ratio (WHR). Start by measuring your waist at its narrowest point when your stomach is relaxed. Then measure your hips at their widest point. Now divide your waist measurement by your hip measurement to get your WHR.

Women should have a WHR of no more than 0.80; for men, it should be no more than 0.95. For more information about the importance of these numbers and what to do if they are too high, see Step 6.

REDalert !

YOUR WAISTLINE

Losing abdominal fat can dramatically lower your risk of having a stroke or mini-stroke. When scientists in Germany studied 379 people who had had a stroke or mini-stroke, and then compared them with 758 people in the same age and sex groups, they found that measures of abdominal fat were strongly associated with the risk of an attack.

Men with a waist circumference greater than 40 in (101 cm) and women whose waists measured more than 35 in (88 cm) had a four-fold increased risk of strokes compared with those with normal waist sizes. Similarly, people with the highest waist-to-hip ratio (over 0.97 for men or 0.84 for women) ran almost eight times the risk compared with those with the lowest WHR (less than 0.92 for men or 0.78 for women).

TAKE YOUR PULSE

You can assess your general level of fitness simply by measuring your pulse rate while you are at rest. In one study of nearly 130,000 post-menopausal women who had no history of heart problems, those with the lowest resting pulse rate (fewer than 62 beats a minute) were significantly less likely to have a heart attack or die of coronary artery disease within the following eight years than those with the highest rate (more than 76 beats a minute). A similar association between pulse rate and cardiovascular risk has been demonstrated in studies involving men.

To check your resting pulse rate, make sure that you can see a clock or watch with a second hand. Then feel the inside of your wrist about two fingers' breadth above the base of your thumb, or in the hollow on one side

You can get a good idea of your general fitness level simply by measuring your pulse rate when at rest.

of your windpipe, just under your jawbone, at the level of your Adam's apple (see photograph). While looking at the second hand of the clock or watch, count the number of heart beats you can feel in 15 seconds. Multiply the figure you arrive at by four to get the number of heart beats per minute—this is your pulse rate.

Check your pulse rate when you are still and calm. An ideal time is right after you wake up, as long as you haven't just been seriously startled by a loud alarm clock. As a guide, the average adult resting pulse rate is about 75 beats a minute for a woman and 70 for a man. Note down your current rate in your diary. As you get fitter, it should decrease.

OTHER POINTS TO NOTE

As mentioned earlier, smoking sends your cardiovascular risk spiraling. The risk posed by smoking increases with age and subsides only after five years have elapsed since the person kicked the habit. So if you do smoke, you need to recognize that smoking is a serious risk factor. For the sake of your heart and brain, you would be wise to take steps to give it up. See Step 8 for some sound quitting strategies.

Surprisingly, scientific studies have also established a significant link between gum disease and the risk of experiencing a heart attack or stroke. So be on the alert for red, swollen or bleeding gums—gums that bleed when you brush your teeth represent an early sign of gum disease. You have a greater risk of gum disease if you smoke, grind your teeth or are under stress. Good dental care will benefit your general health, so ensure that you have regular checkups.

Robert Cutter

A lucky escape

Robert Cutter, who runs a civil engineering business, was working on some machinery in a quarry when he experienced unusual, cramp-like pains across his chest. "I felt really unwell and my face was hot and sweaty," he says, "but I didn't have a clue what was going on. The pains got so bad that I went home and finally managed to get upstairs - but then I dropped to the floor. I phoned my sister, who dialed 911."

When the ambulance arrived 20 minutes later, an ECG (electrocardiogram) confirmed that Robert had had a heart attack. It was more than an hour since the onset of his symptoms, and the nearest hospital was 45 minutes away. But Robert was lucky: The ambulance crew had just started to carry a clot-busting drug, and he was the first person in the new scheme to receive the drug outside of the hospital.

The effect was remarkable. "As soon as they gave me the drug I was completely okay," says Robert.

Amazingly, he suffered no damage to his heart and went home a few days later. A later test revealed that one of his coronary arteries was kinked - probably a condition he was born with - and a device called a stent was inserted to hold the artery open.

"Now I'm careful to eat the right things: more fish, greens and salads. Eating is crucial - what you eat is what you are."

But Robert also acknowledges that before the attack, his blood pressure had been a little high. He didn't relax or exercise very much, and his diet was unhealthy.

"Now I'm careful to eat the right things: more fish, greens and salads. Eating is crucial - what you eat is what you are. And I smoked sometimes before, but I've stopped that now. I avoid cigarettes like the plague."

Since adopting his new regime, his general health has improved. "I go walking and cycling now too. I still have a busy lifestyle running my own business. It is stressful, but I enjoy it and I try not to worry so much."

your body's fuel

An unhealthy diet can increase your risk of heart attacks and strokes. So it is important to keep an eye on what you eat and drink. Answer the questions below and record your score. When you get to the end, add up all the figures to find out whether your drinks, snacks and meals help to protect you ("low" risk), have a "moderate" but not especially helpful effect or could be raising your cardiovascular risk ("increased" risk).

Which would you prefer as a quick snack?

- An apple, banana or handful of grapes   15
- Carrot sticks with a dip   10
- A handful of nuts – salted   5
                                    – natural   10
- Chips, a cookie or a slice of cake   0

How many portions of oily fish do you eat per week?

(Salmon, trout and mackerel are examples of oily fish.)

- 0   0
- 1   10
- 2–4   15

Women who are or plan to become pregnant are advised not to have more than 2 portions of oily fish per week; high concentrations of mercury from ocean pollution may be present in the body fats of some oily fish, representing a potential danger, through the mother, to the health of an unborn child.

How many times a week do you eat packaged meals or take-out?

- 0   15
- 1   5
- More than 1   0

How many portions of the following do you have in an average week?

Sausages, pies, burgers, hot dogs, kebabs or fatty meats such as bacon

- 0   15
- 1   5
- More than 1   0

On average, how often do you eat cakes, pastries, cookies or chips?

- Most days   0
- 2–3 times a week   5
- Once a week or less   15

What kind of fat do you tend to cook with?

- Butter, lard or drippings   0
- Vegetable oils, such as canola   5
- Olive oil   15

Which of these cooking methods do you use most often?

- Deep frying   0
- Pan frying   5
- Broiling, poaching, baking or steaming   15

Which is closest to your usual breakfast?

- Nothing—I never eat before mid-morning — 0
- A coffee and pastry on the way to work — 0
- The works: bacon, eggs and sausages — 0
- Whole wheat toast and jam — 5
- Muesli/high-fiber cereal such as Weetabix, with fresh fruit — 10
- Oatmeal or fruit with low-fat yogurt — 15

Do you check food labels for saturated, hydrogenated and trans fats (the "bad" ones), then make choices that way?

- Yes, always — 15
- Sometimes — 5
- Never — 0

Do you check labels for salt content and make choices that way?

- Yes, usually — 10
- Sometimes — 5
- Never — 0

Nobody should be eating more than 2400 mg of sodium a day, so avoid foods with high sodium content and look in instead for those with less than 140 mg (or even better, 5 mg) per serving.

Which of these is the closest to your drinking pattern?

- Teetotal—no alcohol or less than one drink per month — 10
- Moderate drinking—2–14 servings a week for women, 3–21 servings a week for men — 15
- Excess drinking—more than 14 servings a week for women, more than 21 servings a week for men — 0
- Binge drinking—regularly consuming 6 or more servings in a single session — 0

A 5-ounce (142 mL) glass of wine, 12 ounces (340 mL) of beer or 1.5 ounces (42.6 mL) of hard liquor is considered a serving.

Do you eat white rice, white pasta, white bread or sugary breakfast cereals?

- Daily — 0
- 3–4 times a week — 5
- Once or twice a week, or less often — 15

ADD UP YOUR TOTAL SCORE

YOUR RISK ASSESSMENT

low	moderate	increased
100 or more	50–99	49 or less

your body's output

There is plenty of evidence that physical activity—or, rather, lack thereof—plays a considerable role in the development of cardiovascular disease. Getting fit may require extra effort since so many of today's jobs involve sitting for long periods of time. Evenings in front of the television don't help either. So how active is your lifestyle? For the benefit of your heart and arteries, should you be doing more?

Which activities do you do regularly (at least once a week)?
- Go to the gym, run, cycle or play a sport   15
- Enjoy a leisurely walk in the park   10
- Run up the stairs instead of taking the elevator   5
- Reach for the remote control   0

If you work, how much activity do you get in the course of a working day?
- Walk to the photocopier or coffee machine a few times   0
- Make the effort to walk at least part of the way to work,
  or run upstairs a couple of times during the day   5
- At least a third of my working time is spent moving around 10
- Manual work, constantly on the go   15

On average, how many hours a day do you spend not sitting or lying down?
- 6 or more   15
- 3–5   5
- Fewer than 3   0

Score 5 points for each hour's activity you do during an average week:
- Housework   ---
- Gardening   ---
- DIY projects, such as home repair   ---
- Walking the dog   ---
- Cleaning the car   ---

On average, how much exercise do you get each week that makes you out of breath?
- At least 30 minutes, five days a week   15
- Two hours or less in total   5
- None   0

How many hours a week do you spend watching television?
- 15 or more   0
- 5–14   5
- Fewer than 5   15

Can you climb two standard flights of stairs without getting out of breath?
- Yes, running   15
- Yes, walking pace   10
- No   0

Would people describe you as fidgety?
- Yes   10
- No   0

Your ideal day off would be spent doing which of the following?
- Lying in front of the television and raiding the fridge occasionally   0
- Relaxing with a good book and spending time with your family   5
- Taking a walk in the park and meeting friends for lunch   10
- Sailing, hiking, fencing or a similar energetic activity   15

Would you run to catch a bus or train that was about to leave rather than wait for the next one?
- Yes   10
- No   0

ADD UP YOUR TOTAL SCORE

YOUR RISK ASSESSMENT

low	moderate	increased
60 or more	36–59	35 or less

your work

Stress at work can affect your chances of developing cardiovascular disease. Answer yes or no to the following questions to assess your risk (skip this section if you are self-employed, unemployed or retired).

Do you regularly feel under pressure at work?
Do you feel your immediate boss is sometimes unfair?
Do you commute to work by public transport?
Do you regularly work longer than 45 hours per week?
Do you take work home more than once a month?
Do you answer work emails or phone calls away from the office?

ADD UP THE NUMBER OF "YES" ANSWERS

YOUR RISK ASSESSMENT

low	moderate	increased
0–2	3–4	5–6

your daily surroundings

Your cardiovascular risk can be affected by a variety of factors in your environment, from the people you share your home with to the air you breathe. Answer yes or no to the following questions:

Do you live with someone who smokes?
Do you live within earshot of a main road?
Do you regularly walk or cycle in heavy traffic?
Is your home or workplace often noisy?
Does most of your food come in plastic packaging?
Most days, do you only see the people you work with?

ADD UP THE NUMBER OF "YES" ANSWERS

YOUR RISK ASSESSMENT

low	moderate	increased
0–2	3–4	5–6

your nights

How many hours of sleep do you usually get at night?
- 5 or less — 0
- 6 to 8 — 15
- 9 or more — 0

Which most closely describes your usual sleeping pattern:
- I sleep soundly all night — 15
- I may wake up once to go to the bathroom, but fall asleep again easily — 15
- I have trouble falling asleep but sleep soundly the rest of the night — 5
- I tend to wake several times in the night and have difficulty getting back to sleep — 0
- I wake up early in the morning and it's pointless trying to sleep again — 0

During the day do you regularly:
- Wake up still feeling tired — 0
- Feel tired or sleepy most of the day — 0
- Tend to drop off unexpectedly when you sit quietly — 0
- Take a siesta — 10

Do you snore?
(Answer yes if your partner or children say you do, even if you don't believe it.)
- Yes — 0
- No — 15

Do you sleep in the same room as a snorer?
- Yes   0
- No   10

ADD UP YOUR TOTAL SCORE [   ]

YOUR RISK ASSESSMENT

low	moderate	increased
low	**moderate**	**increased**
more than 35	16–34	up to 15

the people around you

Which of these best describes your home life?
- Stressful   0
- Dull   0
- Supportive   15
- Friendly chaos   10

If you have a romantic relationship, would you describe it as mainly:
- Happy and supportive   15
- A bit of a compromise   5
- Tense and argumentative   0
- Stressful and unhappy   0

How many friends do you have in whom you can confide?
- None   0
- 1–2   5
- 3–5   10
- More than 5   15

Are you friendly with at least one neighbor?
- Yes   10
- No   0

How many hugs did you share on an average day this week?
- None   0
- 1–3   5
- 4 or more   15

ADD UP YOUR TOTAL SCORE [   ]

YOUR RISK ASSESSMENT

low	moderate	increased
low	**moderate**	**increased**
40 or more	16–39	less than 15

your inner life

The way you feel, your habits, attitudes and interests all play a role in your risk of experiencing cardiovascular disease. Discover how your interaction with life could be adding to—or protecting you from—the risk of heart attacks and strokes.

Does worrying about money sometimes keep you awake at night?
- Yes   0
- No   10

Do you make sure you have some time to relax every day, if only for a few minutes?
- Yes   15
- No   0

How would you describe your general health?
- Pretty good   15
- Just a few niggling problems   10
- I have a number of health problems that interfere with my life   0

Do you ever experience panic attacks where you get anxious, feel shaky and your heart beats very fast?
- Yes   0
- No   5

Do you often feel lonely?
- Yes   0
- No   10

Do you often get irritable or uncontrollably angry?
- Yes   0
- No   10

Do you sometimes feel there's no point trying to make things better?
- Yes   0
- No   10

Do you have a hobby or interest that takes you out of the house, at least once a week?
- Yes   15
- No   0

Do you regularly pursue interests that stimulate your mind (such as doing crosswords, reading books, learning a language, playing chess)?
- Yes   15
- No   0

Would people describe you as having a good sense of humor?
- Yes   15
- No   0

How do you feel the next five years are likely to turn out?
- I'm excited about them   15
- I know I'll cope with any problems   10
- Thinking about the future makes me anxious   0

ADD UP YOUR TOTAL SCORE

YOUR RISK ASSESSMENT

low	moderate	increased
80 or more	29–79	less then 30

your happiness

How often during the past week have you felt the following emotions?
- I felt hopeful about the future
- I was happy
- I enjoyed life
- I felt that I was just as good as other people

For each of the four items, score as follows:
0 = rarely or none of the time (less than 1 day during the week)
1 = some or a little of the time (1-2 days a week)
2 = occasionally or a moderate amount of the time (3-4 days a week)
3 = most or all of the time (5-7 days a week)
If you're not sure, try recording your feelings at bedtime each day next week.

YOUR RISK ASSESSMENT
Add up your total score for all four items. The maximum possible is 12, a generally happy state of mind, and the minimum 0, not happy at all. The higher your score, the more protection you have against cardiovascular disease.

turning point
Now you have put your life under the microscope and uncovered a rich seam of information—not only about your health, but also about your personality, feelings and behavior. The more frequently you scored moderate or high in the risk assessments, the more necessary it is to take action now and lower your risk. In Step 4, you will discover how to initiate changes that will help you to reach your goal of a healthy heart and healthy arteries.

self-defense plan
STEP
4

NOW THAT YOU'VE LEARNED MORE ABOUT THE LINKS BETWEEN LIFESTYLE CHOICES AND GOOD HEALTH, YOU CAN USE THIS INSIGHT TO HELP YOU DEVISE A PRACTICAL APPROACH TO CUTTING THE RISK OF STROKES, HEART DISEASE AND OTHER RELATED CONDITIONS.

Make your
personal plan

If you have considered all the issues covered in Step 3, completed the questionnaires and taken stock of the results, you should now be able to make a fair assessment of how your lifestyle might be affecting your risk of developing cardiovascular disease. You should also have discovered which categories of risk are most relevant to you — whether they are an expanding waistline, unbalanced diet, stressful job or regular loss of sleep.

Some of the information revealed in Step 3 may have surprised you. Did you know, for example, that gum disease is a risk factor for heart attacks? Or that housework and gardening can protect your arteries? Or that simply sitting for long periods, or watching television for hours on end, are risk factors for cardiovascular disease in their own right?

FIGHTING BACK

Apart from your age and gender, you have the power to modify every single one of the risk factors identified in Step 3. You may need to enlist the help of your doctor to combat some of them. Others you'll be able to tackle yourself as you develop your long-term strategic plan to protect against heart attacks, strokes and the atherosclerosis (artery damage) that usually causes them.

THE POWER OF PLEASURE

What you'll also discover is the importance of emotional well-being and how happiness, underpinned by supportive relationships and stimulating interests, holds a vital key to good health. And you'll find out how you can reduce your cardiovascular risk by identifying the elements of your own life that bring you pleasure and enjoyment—be they hobbies that you're passionate about, or special people who make you happy.

think yourself well

How healthy you believe yourself to be may have a crucial bearing on your life expectancy. In one research study, a group of hotel cleaners—many of whom perceived themselves as inactive and unfit—were asked to listen to a presentation about the ways in which their daily cleaning routine provided them with an excellent physical workout. They were given information sheets showing how many calories they used while performing such tasks as vacuuming a staircase or cleaning a bathroom. A few weeks later, the workers had lost an average of 2lb in weight, reduced their blood pressure levels and achieved some reduction in body mass index (BMI) and body fat—yet none of them had changed their diet or exercise habits at all.

ADDED HEALTH BENEFITS

Looking after the health of your arteries will benefit your general physical and mental health, and give you a good chance of avoiding other, linked conditions such as peripheral arterial disease and diabetes. As you grow older, having healthier arteries will help to preserve your teeth, eyesight and hearing, and make it less likely that you will develop dementia.

Having healthier arteries will help to preserve your teeth, eyesight and hearing as you grow older.

MOMENT OF TRUTH

While completing the lifestyle questionnaires in Step 3, you may have noted potential health problems that you'd never considered before. Perhaps you were surprised when you measured your BMI (see page 66), or by the amount of abdominal fat you had acquired (see page 67). You may have noticed how breathless you tend to get while climbing stairs—and how little exercise you do. Were you aware how many cigarettes you were smoking? Or did you realize that you never seem to have time to unwind these days and feel edgy and tense?

These are some of the risk factors identified in the Interheart study described in Step 1 (see page 17). It's worth looking back and considering the nine factors that account for 90 percent of all first-time heart attacks.

If you scored "low" in most of the questionnaires, congratulations. Whether you knew it or not, you are doing most things right. But, for most people, there will be something to change, and the following steps make that easy and enjoyable. The most encouraging aspect of all this advice is that you will feel better, younger and fitter once you make a few tweaks.

get a cardiovascular health check

Making an appointment with your doctor is an excellent starting point as you begin to assess the practical ways to address any of the health risks you uncovered in Step 3. This is particularly important if you are over 40 and haven't had your blood pressure or cholesterol checked in the past

An appointment with your doctor is an excellent starting point to address any health risks you've uncovered.

couple of years. If you have several risk factors, you could ask your doctor to carry out a full checkup on the health of your heart, known medically as a cardiovascular risk assessment. Such advice applies if you are a heavy smoker; if your waist measurement exceeds 35 in (88 cm) for a woman, or 40 in (102 cm) for a man; if you have a family history of heart disease or strokes; or if, for any other reason, you are at a higher risk of developing heart disease.

DISCUSS DIABETES

Overweight people who are concerned about developing metabolic syndrome, or "pre-diabetes" (see pages 30–31), should ask their doctor to monitor their urine for sugar and, if necessary, to arrange blood tests to check their blood sugar levels.

About half of those people who are diagnosed with Type 2 diabetes already exhibit signs of cardiovascular disease at the time of diagnosis. Taking action to overcome underlying problems such as obesity could help to reduce your risks of both problems.

SECRET weapon

GENETIC COUNSELORS

Coronary heart disease (CHD) tends to run in families, though your risk is greatly reduced if you are healthy and fit. Certain rare inherited heart conditions are more dangerous, however, as they develop in young people regardless of lifestyle, are often symptomless and can cause sudden cardiac death. Causes of sudden cardiac death include Brugada syndrome, long QT syndrome and pre-excitation syndrome. All involve genetic and/or structural abnormalities that lead to potentially fatal alternations in heart rhythm. Unfortunately, they are rarely diagnosed prior to a crisis.

If your family history shows one of the ailments mentioned above, you might consider speaking with a genetic counselor about being tested. For more information, visit the National Society of Genetic Counselors (nsgc.org) or American Board of Genetic Counselors (abgc.net) if you're in the United States, or the Canadian Association of Genetic Counsellors at cagc-accg.ca.

YOUR CALCIUM SCORE

One of the tools doctors may use to diagnose heart disease is an EBCT (electron beam computed tomography) scan. The scan can reveal information about soft tissues as well as bones, which means that it may be used to examine internal organs such as your heart. EBCT scans can identify and measure calcium deposits that are found in a buildup of hard plaque on artery walls. If you have no calcium, you can assume that your risk of having a heart attack is very low. However, most people develop some plaques containing calcium in their arteries as they age, so the older you are, the less likely you are to have a zero score. A mid-range score indicates that serious measures are required to reduce cardiovascular risk. A high coronary calcium score means that you almost certainly have coronary heart disease.

PROTECTIVE MEASURES

If your doctor tells you that you have a moderate or high risk of developing cardiovascular disease, he or she may recommend that you try to improve your diet, do more exercise, set a target for weight loss and cut down on stress. Advice on all these aspects of healthier living are covered in future steps in this book, as are plenty of tips to help make changing habits more fun. If you smoke, you should tackle this as your top priority and, if necessary, enlist your doctor's help to find the therapy or medication that will help you quit. All of these measures will also help to lower your blood pressure.

If you are at high risk (that is, you have a 20 percent or greater chance of developing cardiovascular disease over the next ten years), you may be prescribed statins to reduce cholesterol levels and, possibly, drugs to reduce blood pressure or treat diabetes. In this case, the measures outlined in *Conquering Heart Attacks & Strokes* will be an added bonus. The invaluable information in the rest of this book will enable you to keep your treatment on target, and even help you reduce your medication. You might eventually be able to stop taking the tablets altogether.

Smoking is such a major risk factor that you should make it your top priority to quit.

your scores and your choices

The results you obtained from completing the questionnaires in Step 3 reveal which factors are contributing most strongly to your risk of having a heart attack or stroke. You need to focus attention on any instance where you scored "moderate" or "increased." Make a list of the problem areas identified by the questionnaires, then follow the guide below to find practical advice and imaginative strategies for tackling them.

your body individual risk factors:

- **Excess weight**
- **Abdominal fat**
- **Smoking**
- **High resting pulse rate**
- **Gum disease**

WHERE TO FIND HELP

If you need to lose weight, Step 5 will help you to make a thorough reassessment of your diet and provides a multitude of tips on how to make the small changes that will yield large benefits for your weight.

Step 6 allows you to figure out what's causing you to put on weight, and takes a long hard look at the dangers posed by processed food and junk food. It also describes tactics for resisting temptation and gives advice on where to go for expert professional help.

If you are carrying too much abdominal fat, you'll know that it's notoriously difficult to lose. Step 6 explains how a two-pronged attack of diet and exercise really does work—even if the enemy has gained a lot of ground—and includes a list of those foods that can actually protect you against putting on too much fat around your middle.

Step 7 is full of ideas for getting pleasure out of physical exertion, even if exercise is not your favorite thing. It also has tips for building up cardiovascular strength and stamina.

A high pulse rate when you are at rest tends to indicate a lack of fitness. Step 7 sets out strategies for getting active that can be incorporated with ease into everyday life, without the need to spend long sessions in the gym. It is worth noting that a trained athlete can have a pulse rate as low as 40 beats per minute, while the average resting heart rate for an adult is between 60 and 100 beats per minute.

If you are a smoker, you have probably tried to kick the habit at least once. It's a difficult thing to do if you're living a fast-paced life. But did you know that, however much you smoke, halving that number of cigarettes also reduces your risk by half? In Step 8 you will learn how to shore up your willpower with a combination of physical and psychological tactics. See the Resources section (page 240) for useful helplines. (Studies have shown that people who have support—medical, emotional or both—are much more likely to succeed in giving up smoking.)

Gum disease increases your risk of experiencing heart disease or strokes. In Step 8 you will find out how to spot the early signs of gum disease and learn what you need to do to prevent it.

your body's fuel individual risk factors:

- **Not enough fruit or vegetables**
- **Too many saturated or trans fats**
- **Not enough oily fish**
- **Too many processed or junk foods**
- **Too many snacks**
- **Cooking unhealthily**
- **Too much salt**
- **Too much alcohol**
- **Too many refined carbohydrates**

WHERE TO FIND HELP

Your diet has a major impact on the condition of your arteries. Step 5 identifies the best foods for healthy arteries and those to avoid. Also explained is the latest research into why fruit, vegetables and certain types of fat provide potent protection against heart attacks and strokes. Cutting down on sodium, or salt, is key in the battle against high blood pressure, but it's not just the salt we add to food ourselves that should concern us; anything from canned soup to cookies can also contain hidden salt.

small change, big gain

According to researchers in the UK, if everyone in that country simply replaced an unhealthy daily snack (a chocolate bar, a bag of chips, a pastry) with a healthy one (a piece of fresh or dried fruit, raw vegetables, unsalted nuts or seeds), it could lead to the prevention of nearly 6,000 deaths from cardiovascular disease each year. Scientists at the University of Liverpool have calculated that each Briton would consume around 4.4 g less saturated fat per day, leading to 2,400 fewer deaths from coronary artery disease and 425 fewer deaths from strokes. Clearly, good nutrition is a key to better living no matter where you live.

your body's output individual risk factors:

- **Sedentary job and too much sitting in general**
- **Too much television**
- **Not enough exercise**
- **General lack of fitness**
- **Not enough walking**

WHERE TO FIND HELP

Step 7 shows you how to enjoy getting into shape. Even if you are taking up exercise for the first time later in life, there are gentle activities to benefit your circulation, increase your muscular strength and help you to live longer. And you'll learn how everyday activities, including gardening and housework, burn calories and help you keep fit.

SECRET weapon

TAKE THE STAIRS

Even a change as simple as climbing up and down the stairs at work instead of using the elevator could improve your chances of living longer, according to researchers in Switzerland. A team from the University of Geneva asked 69 university employees—who each habitually did less than two hours of exercise a week—to abandon the elevator and to use the stairs. Over a period of 12 weeks, the volunteers climbed or descended on average 23 flights of stairs a day (up from five a day before the study). Their lung capacity, blood pressure, waist measurements and cholesterol levels all improved, reducing their risk of premature death by about 15 percent.

Tear yourself away
from the box.

Ray Chadd

How I changed my lifestyle

Turning 50 had a special but serious significance for Ray
Chadd. "I felt perfectly fit and healthy, but I couldn't help
remembering that my father had died suddenly of a heart attack
at the age of 56. That was a terrible shock. I started
wondering if I might be vulnerable in my fifties, too."

What especially concerned him, too, was that his youngest
daughter was only three years old. "My wife wanted me to go
for a checkup. I never went to the doctor - I was never sick.
But she said something like, 'What would we do without you?'
and that was enough. I made an appointment with the doctor."

The doctor found that Ray's blood pressure was, indeed, on
the high side and advised him to be careful with his diet and
cut down on salt. He began to eat more fruit and vegetables,
less meat and fewer sweets. "You may laugh, but plain yogurt
mixed with fresh fruit became my favorite food. I felt better
and I had more energy, too. We started playing tennis, which
was fun and relaxing. That was good because it was a
stressful time. I was director of the English department at a
local college that was going through a lot of changes."

**"Plain yogurt mixed with chopped-up fresh fruit
became a favorite food. I felt better and I had
more energy too."**

Ray was also referred to a cardiologist and was told that
he had an irregular heartbeat, too. "That was an added reason
to keep my weight and blood pressure under control."

Now 66 and semi-retired, Ray still has regular checkups,
but feels perfectly fit and has successfully avoided the
statins that many of his contemporaries have to take.

For that he thanks his lifestyle tweaks: a moderate diet,
plus regular exercise from going up and down the many stairs
at his home and walking his son's dog. He was also pleased to
note a recent Dutch study, which concluded that a little wine
daily is even better protection against heart attacks than
being a teetotaler. "I certainly enjoy red wine," says Ray,
"but I only drink about half a glass a day."

your work individual factors:

- **Pressure at work**
- **Unfair boss**
- **Commuting**
- **Long hours**
- **Taking work home**
- **Work emails or phone calls away from the office**

WHERE TO FIND HELP

If you are an office worker, you probably find that, even when you manage to escape from your desk, someone tries to reach you by cell phone. Some days it seems impossible to distance yourself from work obligations. Step 9 outlines some stress management techniques and explains why it's so important to set yourself limits and learn to switch off from work.

your daily surroundings
individual risk factors:

- **Living with a smoker**
- **Living near a main road**
- **Exposure to heavy traffic**
- **Exposure to loud noise**
- **Dealing with domestic stress**
- **Living alone**

WHERE TO FIND HELP

Smoking endangers not only your own health, but the health of those around you. Step 8 offers effective strategies for breaking the habit. If there is another smoker in the family or among your group of friends, see if you can make a pact to quit together.

SECRETweapon

EARPLUGS

Exposure to the din of modern life may increase an individual's risk of heart disease. Studies of car assembly workers suggests that continuous exposure to noise increases blood pressure, but that using earplugs can largely prevent this. Conversely, by protecting your arteries, you will also protect your hearing, since cardiovascular disease can clog the tiny arteries that feed the delicate hearing mechanisms of the inner ear. Whatever the source of noise in your life—airplanes, traffic, road work or machinery—using a pair of earplugs is a cheap and easy way to take care of your hearing, and your heart.

Noise pollution can be particularly difficult to avoid if you live or work in an urban area or work around noisy machines. Step 8 includes advice on how to protect yourself from noise pollution and the toxic substances that lurk in your environment.

your nights individual risk factors:

- Snoring
- Sleeping with a snorer
- Too little sleep—or too much
- Disturbed sleep
- Daytime sleepiness

WHERE TO FIND HELP

Sleep deprivation exerts a serious toll on our bodies. Simply stated, people who sleep better live longer. In Step 9 you will find expert advice on how to sleep easy, as well as advice on how to deal with snoring.

your inner life individual factors:

- Financial worries
- Insufficient relaxation
- Feeling unhealthy
- Panic attacks
- Loneliness
- Hopelessness or pessimism
- Lack of interests
- Inadequate mental stimulation
- Poor sense of humour

WHERE TO FIND HELP

Most of us assume that external things are what make us happy. But Step 9 dispels this myth and explains that the key to a full and healthy life is finding the strategy that suits you.

the people around you
Individual risk factors:

- Stressful home life
- Unstimulating home life
- Unsupportive relationships
- Lack of friends
- Isolation from neighbors

WHERE TO FIND HELP

Chronic stress, isolation and lack of support can all accelerate the progress of atherosclerosis. No matter what your age, where you live or whether you have a job, partner or children, there are things you can do to turn your life around. Laughter, friendship and a range of stimulating interests are golden tickets to better health and a better quality of life. Find out more in Step 9.

it's time to talk tactics

Don't try to fix everything at once. If you suddenly decide that you want to lose 10 lb in two weeks, immediately embark on a major exercise program and revolutionize your eating habits, you probably won't get far before you become discouraged and give up (especially if you also need to tackle other tough issues such as quitting smoking, dealing with a difficult boss or deciding what to do about an unhappy relationship).

THE KEY TO SUCCESS

To boost your confidence and maintain your motivation, start by making changes that are minor but sustainable. Here are some ideas for small changes that will make a big difference.

ONE STEP AT A TIME
- Make an appointment with your doctor or dentist.
- Buy olive oil instead of your usual cooking oil.
- Use the stairs instead of the elevator at work.
- Swap one unhealthy snack today for a piece of fruit.
- Eat fish instead of meat for dinner tonight.
- Leave work on time one day this week.
- Take the salt shaker off the table.
- Give your partner a hug for no reason.
- Go for a half-hour stroll instead of watching television.
- Invite your neighbor over for coffee.

SET SMART GOALS

If you are determined to make your plan work and maintain it, you will need to define and prioritize your goals. For example, based on what you learned in Step 3, choose one element of your life associated with a high risk of cardiovascular disease, read the relevant information here and decide on the most important changes that you need to make. Set your targets, write them down and give yourself a timeframe for achieving them.

For example, if you need to lose 20 lb to achieve your ideal weight, it is clear that this will take several months. So set an interim goal, such as losing 5 lb by the end of next month. Similarly, if you acknowledge that your diet has many shortcomings, don't imagine that you can fix everything in a few days. Pick small, specific targets, such as foregoing a microwavable meal or take-out once a week and making one or two home-cooked meals from scratch using healthy ingredients. Or take healthy snacks to work instead of buying chocolate bars and chips from a vending machine or convenience store.

Make the process of changing to a healthier lifestyle as much fun as you can. For instance, for every 2 lb you lose, reward yourself in some way. Take a weekend off, buy something special, look up old friends—and plan for a future that features a healthier, happier you.

Set an interim goal, don't imagine that you can put everything right in a few days.

BE REALISTIC ...

One thing you will be aware of by now is that warding off heart attacks and strokes is not a short-term maneuver like a crash diet. If the many small changes you are contemplating are going to keep you protected for the rest of your life, you need to work them into your everyday routine. Only then will you have the motivation to keep them going.

... AND PRAGMATIC

Another important element of the process is to decide what you can change. It's no good telling your boss that you refuse to work late ever again, but you can quietly look around for a new job, or retrain so you can move to a company that makes fewer demands on your personal life. Or you might decide to use some relaxing techniques to reduce stress related to overworking or a difficult work environment.

If you live next to a main road, you may not be in a position to move, but you could buy earplugs to help you get a better night's sleep. Throughout this book, you will find a wealth of advice to help you fend off cardiovascular risks—even though you may not be able to avoid them altogether.

MAINTAIN MOMENTUM

Once you understand what's realistic, you can devise a timetable. You can't alter the habits of a lifetime in a few weeks, but you can start to make changes that will last, and build on them. You will find it useful to keep a running record in a notebook so you can see your successes, or remember what didn't work and try something else.

Take advantage of whatever support is available. Tell your friends that you are quitting smoking and ask for their help. Cajole your partner or children to join you in getting involved in more physical activities. Talk to your doctor if you run into problems with your weight-loss regime. As your doctor knows, by making these healthy changes now, you will be less likely to have dangerous fats attacking your arteries—and you will be less likely to need medication for high blood pressure, high cholesterol or even heart disease in the future.

MUSIC

Learning to play a musical instrument could be good for your heart, say scientists at the University of Oxford in the United Kingdom and the University of Pavia in Italy. They studied breathing and circulation in 24 young people before and while the subjects listened to excerpts of music. Half were trained musicians who had been playing instruments such as the violin, piano, flute, clarinet or bass for several years. The rest had no musical training. The music ranged from slow classical music (Beethoven and Indian raga) to fast-paced rock (the Red Hot Chili Peppers). While the faster and more complex rhythms speeded up breathing and circulation, calmer, more meditative tracks also slowed breathing and heart rate in all participants. However, the effects were strongest on the musicians, who were more used to synchronizing breathing with musical phrases. The scientists suggest that the relaxing and stress-reducing effects of music could be useful in preventing and treating heart disease and strokes.

YOUR PLAN FOR LIFE

In the steps that follow, you will discover the tactics and strategies, the important facts and expert advice, to help keep your cardiovascular system healthy. By targeting the root causes now, you will prolong your life. You have already begun taking charge in ways that work for you.

self-defense plan

STEP 5

DELICIOUS MEALS ADD TO THE ENJOYMENT OF LIFE AND THERE'S NO NEED TO FOREGO THEM TO PROTECT YOUR HEART AND ARTERIES. HEALTHY DIETS OFTEN INCLUDE THE FRESHEST, TASTIEST AND MOST COLORFUL NATURAL FOODS BECAUSE THESE ALL HELP TO BUILD UP RESISTANCE TO CARDIOVASCULAR PROBLEMS.

Discover the
pleasures of healthy
eating

Your eating habits have a crucial influence on your risk of cardiovascular disease. Obesity, high cholesterol and disturbed blood sugar in particular are among the food-related factors underlying heart attacks. But we are all given so much conflicting information about healthy eating that, for those who want to improve their diets, it is difficult to know who to believe or how to start.

HELPING YOU CHOOSE

Step 5 aims to cut through the general confusion about diets to provide clear, accessible advice based on the most authoritative research and expert opinions. You will find out about foods that can wreak havoc on your body, such as saturated fats, salt, refined carbohydrates and sugar. And you will learn about beneficial foods—such as fruit, vegetables, fish and even red wine—that help fight the causes of cardiovascular disease. This advice will help you to make informed choices and add more delicious ingredients to what you eat every day.

MAGIC FOODS

Don't be put off by the thought that you need to change everything. There are enjoyable and simple ways to enhance your diet without self-sacrifice. Eating fresh, natural foods that are full of flavor will encourage you to develop a totally new eating pattern. Building up your dietary defenses in stages will make change easier and help you to adopt eating habits that will benefit your long-term health. In fact, once you have followed this healthy eating plan for a month, you will never look back.

I'm pretty fit, I'm not overweight and I play tennis three times a week. Surely I don't need to worry about what I eat?

An active lifestyle is undoubtedly beneficial to health, but if you want to keep your body in peak condition in the years to come, you will need to give it the right sort of fuel. So it really is in your own interests to find out about foods that will protect your heart and arteries, foods that will help to build and maintain your bones and muscles, and foods that will help to keep your weight down as you get older—and adapt your long-term diet accordingly.

what's wrong with our diets?

People in North America are getting fatter. Part of the reason is that many of us tend to make poor choices—eating processed foods that are high in sugar, refined carbohydrates, salt and unhealthy fats. These also tend to be laden with calories which, for anyone with an inactive lifestyle, are hard to burn off. This spells trouble for our health because it prompts the body to make too much "bad" LDL cholesterol, which, together with other factors such as inflammation, leads to the formation of artery-clogging plaque.

During the past 50 years, more and more of us have come to depend heavily on premade foods and take-out. A scan of the food aisles in any supermarket will reveal how many common items are far from pure and natural. Most are either processed or artificially sweetened, flavored or coloured, or laced with chemical preservatives to keep them from spoiling. And it is worth remembering that, when fresh, raw whole foods are canned, precooked or turned into microwavable meals, many essential vitamins, minerals and nutrients are lost.

CLUES FROM THE PAST

Our bodies are not designed to thrive on processed food. Genetically, we are still hunter-gatherers—as we have been since the late Paleolithic era, or Stone Age, some 40,000 years ago. Yet our diet is completely different from that of our ancestors who ate only natural foods obtained by hunting and foraging. More than 70 percent of energy intake in modern Western diets comes from foods that were unknown in the Stone Age. These include refined carbohydrates such as those in white flour, white bread

Avoid refined
carbohydrates such as
white flour, white bread and
white rice, which have been heavily processed.

and white rice, which have been heavily processed, thereby removing many of their beneficial qualities. Since the modern diet is calorie-dense rather than nutrient-dense, many of us are eating more calories daily than we can use up in physical activity. As a result, we put on weight.

What's more, for most people, affordable food is much more readily available than it has ever been. So unlike our distant ancestors, who struggled to obtain enough food to live on, we often need to limit our intake for our own good health.

"Throughout human evolution, access to food was the major challenge for survival," explains Dr. Stephen O'Rahilly of the University of Cambridge in the United Kingdom. "People who had genetic variants that made them good at storing food as fat would be the most likely to survive and pass the trait on."

This natural tendency rarely led to obesity, because it was balanced by the energy expended in obtaining food. Today we don't have to go out and catch our food. We don't even have to move; the supermarket will deliver it to our door. And what we choose to eat can make matters worse.

This mismatch between our lifestyle and that of our early forebearers is a major factor in the current surge in obesity, hypertension, diabetes, strokes and heart disease. Historical and anthropological studies suggest that our ancestors were largely free of the degenerative cardiovascular diseases that beset many of us today; this also applies to societies in areas of the modern world that are not subject to Western nutritional influences.

THE POWER OF NATURAL FOODS

So what are the benefits of a Stone Age diet? Our ancestors ate game meats, fish, vegetables, berries, other fruit and nuts—in other words, they either speared it or picked it. It was a diet rich in lean protein, vitamins, minerals, monounsaturated and polyunsaturated fats like omega-3 fatty

A high-fat, high-sugar diet not only encourages weight gain but is, to some extent, addictive.

acids (see page 105), fiber and other beneficial plant chemicals. These natural foods contain elements that help to keep our cardiovascular system in good condition. In fact, when volunteers in a recent Swedish study followed a "Stone Age diet" for three weeks, eating as our distant ancestors did, they reduced their average calorie intake by 36 percent, raised protective antioxidant levels in their blood, reduced their systolic pressure (the first number in a blood pressure reading) and had a 72 percent reduction in levels of a harmful clot-promoting factor in their blood. They also lost weight, slimmed their waistlines and reduced their body mass index (BMI). Other research has shown that a Stone Age diet not only lowers blood pressure but also improves insulin sensitivity and lowers levels of C-reactive protein, another risk marker for heart disease (see page 22).

RED alert !

JUNK FOODS MAY HAVE AN ADDICTIVE EFFECT

A diet of junk food may change brain pathways that regulate food intake and program us to eat more. Laboratory tests have shown that animals fed a high-fat, high-sugar diet promptly increase their consumption of this type of food. This strongly suggests that a high-fat, high-sugar diet not only encourages weight gain but is to some extent addictive, making it very difficult to lose weight unless the diet is changed.

UNPROCESSED IS BEST

Following a healthy food plan means selecting whole, unprocessed foods and cutting down on foods that are prepackaged, pre-prepared or highly refined, including sugar and white bread.

The Stone Age diet contains little or no grains or rice, but these are not "bad" foods unless they are over-refined. Eating whole grains and brown rice is, in fact, beneficial because both contain plenty of fiber, which keeps the digestive system healthy and satisfies the appetite, so we need to eat less. Like fruit and vegetables, whole-grain wheat and brown rice are good sources of insoluble fiber. Oats, oat bran and legumes provide soluble fiber, which contributes to heart health by binding to "bad" LDL cholesterol and removing it as waste from the body.

the key to
low blood pressure

Cutting your salt intake is one of the most important changes you can make to keep your blood pressure at a healthy level. One of the benefits of natural rather than processed foods is that they contain little or no sodium chloride (table salt), which is potentially harmful.

Scientists had unexpected confirmation of the damaging effects of salt when they studied an indigenous tribe from South America, the Yanomami, who live in the rainforests of Brazil and Venezuela. The tribe's diet contains little fat, no refined carbohydrates—and no salt. When they die as adults, the Yanomami show no evidence of the cardiovascular disease that is omnipresent in Western civilizations. The average adult blood pressure is lower than 100 systolic (the top number in a reading) and just over 60 diastolic (the second number)—an ideal, healthy level.

WISE UP TO SALT

You don't have to travel to the Amazon to start cutting sodium out of your diet. Reducing daily salt intake by just 0.75g (750mg)—roughly the amount contained in a 40g piece of cheddar cheese—can reduce systolic pressure by 2 to 4 points, and diastolic pressure by 1 to 2 points.

In the United States and Canada, current dietary guidelines call for no more than 2,300 mg a day of sodium for healthy adults, or 1,500 mg for middle-aged and older individuals. Most of us take in much more than that. But it is not salt in cooking, or even the salt that we add to meals, that's the prime culprit. The sodium in processed and pre-prepared foods such as soups, bread, and premade meals accounts for more than three-quarters of our average salt intake.

CHECK FOOD LABELS

If you want to cut down on the amount of salt you consume, it is worth getting into the habit of reading the labels on food packaging before you put items into your shopping cart. Don't be fooled into thinking that

REDalert **!**

THE SNACKING HABIT

Many people munch between meals without a second thought. And studies suggest that when we reach for a snack we don't generally compensate by eating less later on, and that in general we take in more calories than we burn in physical activity. Most snack foods—such as pastries, chips, cookies and sugary drinks, which are just snacks in liquid form—are much more energy-dense than natural unprocessed foods. In Step 6, you will discover how to snack healthily and how to break a bad snacking habit.

Get into the habit of reading the labels on food packaging before you put items into your shopping basket.

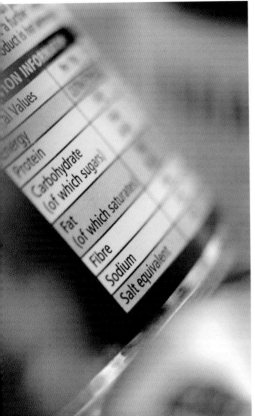

"reduced sodium" means "low sodium". It simply means that the product contains 25 percent less than a comparable product. Anything with more than 1.5g salt or 0.6g sodium per 100g has a high salt content, and it may be worth looking for a lower-salt variety. Low-salt foods have 0.3g salt (0.1g sodium) or less per 100g.

POTASSIUM THE PROTECTOR

Foods that are rich in potassium, such as fruit and vegetables, have the opposite effect to that of salt: They help to lower your blood pressure and consequently reduce your risk of developing cardiovascular disease. Potassium helps to balance the effects of sodium in the body, so maintaining high levels of it has clear health benefits.

Scientists advise that it is the ratio of sodium to potassium in your body that's important. In one study of 2,974 people aged between 30 and 54 whose blood pressure readings were slightly under levels considered high, those with the highest sodium levels in their urine were 20 percent more likely to suffer a heart attack or stroke over the following ten to 15 years than those with the lowest sodium levels. And those individuals with the highest sodium-to-potassium ratio—in other words, far higher levels of sodium than potassium—were 50 percent more likely to experience a stroke, heart attack or another form of cardiovascular disease than those with lower ratios.

FIGHT BACK WITH FRUIT

Since potassium is largely derived from fruit and vegetables, increasing your intake will not only help to counteract the effects of too much salt, but also provide you with nutrients known to have a protective effect against heart attack and stroke. Potassium-rich fruit and vegetables include avocados, bananas, grapes, dates, prunes, raisins, watermelons, leafy green vegetables, broccoli, brussels sprouts, lentils and spinach.

beneficial fats

Most of us know that we eat too much fat and that this increases our risk of obesity, itself a major risk factor for high blood pressure and diabetes. And, as explained in Step 1, obesity boosts the risk of inflammation (see page 22), which scientists now know plays a key role in atherosclerosis, the formation of plaque in our arteries and triggering heart attacks. The solution is not to cut out all fats, however. Some fats are hugely beneficial—the omega-3s in salmon, for instance. The monounsaturated fats in olive oil, nuts and avocados also lower cholesterol and have been shown to reduce inflammation in arteries. Our bodies need fats. Indeed, at least 25 percent of our daily calorie intake should be made up of fats, provided that they are largely unsaturated.

THE LOW-FAT MYTH

Since early studies had indicated that people who ate high-fat diets tended to have more heart attacks, medical experts used to think that following a low-fat diet would help to prevent cardiovascular disease. But more recent research has shown that this approach was flawed. In a 2006 study, the first long-term research of its kind, scientists who had followed 49,000 women for eight years were surprised to find that eating a low-fat diet did not protect against heart attack, stroke or any form of cardiovascular disease.

What had not been appreciated by the earlier experts was that only some types of dietary fat increase the amount of artery-clogging cholesterol in the blood. But the low-fat myth persists. It is still the case that many people who want to lose weight cut back or even cut out all types of fats, including those in olive oil and nuts that actually help to lower cholesterol and safeguard the heart in other ways.

DEFENSEtactics

CUT DOWN ON SATURATED FATS

There are some simple ways to reduce the amount of saturated fat in your diet. The following tips could ward off premature death or heart and health complications due to fat intake:

- Broil, bake or grill foods, especially meat, rather than frying.
- Choose leaner cuts of meat.
- Remove the skin from poultry and trim fat from meat before cooking.
- Choose lower-fat hard cheese. Grate rather than slice hard cheeses, or use smaller amounts of stronger-flavored varieties.
- Use low-fat spreads instead of butter or margarine.
- Before buying packaged foods, check the labels for the saturated-fat content.
- Cut down on your consumption of cakes, candy, desserts and cookies.
- Eat healthier snacks, such as pieces of fresh or dried fruit.
- Switch from full-fat to 2%, 1% or skim milk.

Continued on p. 102 >

Our body's own
good and bad fats

The two most important types of fat in your blood are cholesterol and triglycerides. Regular consumption of protective foods will help to keep them at healthy levels.

CHOLESTEROL – GOOD AND BAD

Your liver, intestines and even your skin create your body's own cholesterol. It binds to proteins and is transported around the body in complex molecules called lipoproteins. Amongst other functions, cholesterol helps to build cell membranes, insulate nerve fibers and make hormones, vitamin D and fat-digesting bile acids.

There are two types of cholesterol. The potentially harmful variety is characterized by low-density lipoproteins (LDLs). Their role is to carry fat from the liver to be used by body cells. LDLs are harmless until they come into contact with unstable molecules in the blood called free radicals, which damage the cholesterol in a process called oxidation. Oxidized LDLs are sucked into the inner linings of artery walls and contribute to the buildup of plaque and inflammation. Excess body fat in the abdominal area, a diet high in saturated fats and lack of activity can all prompt the liver to produce more LDLs.

HEALTHY HDL

"Good" cholesterol is characterised by high-density lipoproteins (HDLs), which travel around the bloodstream mopping up LDLs and transporting them back to the liver for disposal. They may also act as antioxidants, stopping LDLs from causing damage in artery walls. The higher your level of HDL cholesterol, the closer you are to the "natural" cholesterol balance enjoyed in early hunter–gatherer societies, and the lower your risk of having blocked arteries that could prompt a heart attack or stroke.

PROTECTIVE FOODS: Unsaturated fats—from plants, fish and nuts—can lower LDL and raise HDL levels. Omega-3 fats from oily fish such as salmon, walnuts and canola oil are particularly good at raising HDL levels—as is soluble fiber, found in whole grains, fruit such as grapes, brown rice and lentils.

TRIGLYCERIDES

Triglycerides are fats that collect excess calories from the food we eat and speed them away to fat cells for storage. Then, when our bodies need extra energy between meals, stored calories are released. If you eat more calories than you burn off through activity, your triglyceride levels will rise. Levels tend to be high in obese people and those with diabetes or metabolic syndrome, and are raised by consumption of fatty or sugary foods or excess alcohol. High levels of triglycerides are linked to an increased risk of cardiovascular disease, especially in women.

PROTECTIVE FOODS: Unsaturated fats (particularly monounsaturated fat from oils such as olive and canola); fruit (especially citrus) and vegetables; whole grains; and omega-3 fatty acids in fish such as sardines, mackerel and herring.

"DO I NEED TO HAVE TESTS?"

Some people are more at risk of high cholesterol and high triglycerides than others, so being thin and eating healthily doesn't necessarily protect you. There are few physical clues or symptoms linked to the levels of these fats in your bloodstream, which is why it is important that people in any of the groups below should ask their doctor for a cholesterol and triglyceride test:

- Anyone over 40.
- People with established cardiovascular disease—for example, a history of angina, heart attacks, strokes or peripheral vascular disease.
- People with a close family history (parents or siblings) of heart disease or strokes at a young age.
- Anyone—even children—with family members who have a hereditary cholesterol disorder called familial hypercholesterolemia.
- People with risk factors for cardiovascular disease, such as diabetes, high blood pressure, smoking or obesity.

Cholesterol and triglycerides are measured in millimoles per litre (mmol/L) in countries like Canada and the UK, or in milligrams per decilitre (mg/dL) in the US. Generally, ideal targets are: 200 mg/DL (5.2 mmol/L) total cholesterol, with HDL below 130 mg/DL (3.5 mmol/L) and HDL above 40 mg/dL (1.0 mmol/L for men and 1.2 for women). In those with diabetes or high blood pressure, the total should be 154 mg/dL (4.0 mmol/L) or less with an LDL of 77 mg/dL (2.0 mmol/L) or less. For triglycerides, a normal reading is less than 150 mg/dL (1.7 mmol/L). Over 200 mg/dL (2.0 mmol/L) is high and over 500mg/dL (4.5 mmol/L) very high.

If the tests reveal high levels of harmful fats in your blood, your doctor will advise you to cut down on saturated fats and get more exercise. There is some simple advice on how to do this in the following steps. If your cholesterol levels remain high, you may be prescribed cholesterol-lowering statin drugs (which also reduce harmful inflammation).

fats in meat, poultry and fish

A serving size is 2¾ oz (75 g) unless otherwise indicated.

TOTAL FAT IN GRAMS ■   **SATURATED FAT** ■

MEAT
regular minced beef, raw
extra-lean minced beef, raw
pork chop, grilled
ham
1 slice bacon
sirloin steak, grilled
steak, round/rump, grilled

POULTRY
1 chicken breast (5½ oz/150 g), with ½ skin, roast
1 chicken breast (5½ oz/150 g), skinless, roast
roast turkey (5½ oz/150 g), light meat
roast turkey (5½ oz/150 g), dark meat

FISH
salmon, grilled
swordfish, grilled
fresh tuna, grilled
tuna, canned in oil
tuna, canned in water

0g   5g   10g   15g

harmful fats

The type of fat that is particularly damaging to the health of your arteries is saturated fat. It is found mostly in foods derived from animals—fatty cuts of meat, butter, lard, cheese, whole milk and other dairy products—and is generally solid at room temperature. It is also often present in cookies, cakes, pastries, pies, burgers, sausages, chips, french fries and many pre-prepared microwavable meals and deep-fried take-out.

Most of the "bad" LDL cholesterol in our bloodstream is made by the liver from saturated fats in our diet. Although people used to worry about eating eggs because they contain dietary cholesterol, it is our saturated fat

My doctor says my cholesterol level is too high. Should I use a cholesterol-lowering spread?

It might help, but cholesterol-lowering spreads are not routinely recommended for people who have no other signs of cardiovascular disease. Many spreads, yogurt-type drinks and soft cheeses contain added plant chemicals called sterols and stanols, the plant equivalents of cholesterol in humans. They reduce the uptake of cholesterol from the intestines, and this has been shown to reduce levels of total and "bad" LDL cholesterol. However, although foods containing these plant chemicals may help to lower your cholesterol, it is still not clear whether they can reduce your risk of developing cardiovascular disease.

intake, not how much cholesterol we eat, that is mainly responsible for high blood cholesterol levels. On average, about 40 percent of the energy we get from fats comes from saturated fats—and that is much too high.

BEWARE TRANS FATS

Trans fatty acids, or trans fats, are synthetic ingredients found in many margarines, spreads and products such as cakes, pastries, cookies, candy and pre-prepared meals. In recent times, consumption of trans fats has been linked with the increased prevalence of heart attacks and strokes. One Dutch study suggested that cutting out trans fats altogether from our food supply, even if they were replaced by natural vegetable oils, would prevent about 100,000 deaths per year.

Trans fats are chemical by-products of an industrial process called hydrogenation. While experimenting with hydrogen molecules, chemists discovered that they could turn liquid vegetable oil into a solid at room temperature. It seemed like a golden opportunity. Why not use this process to produce cheap and accessible alternatives to products known to be high in unhealthy saturated fats, such as butter and lard? We know now that, far from being a healthier option, these artificially hardened fats behave in the body just like—or possibly worse than—saturated fats.

As evidence against trans fats grows, many North American manufacturers have removed them from their products, while some cities have banned them from restaurants altogether. In Canada, it is compulsory to label products that contain them. When buying packaged food, look for the words "hydrogenated" or "partially hydrogenated" fats on the list of ingredients—if they're in there, they must be declared. If you find them, do your arteries a favor and put the product back on the shelf.

choose unsaturated...

There is every reason to switch to unsaturated fats if you care about the health of your cardiovascular system. The two types, monounsaturated and polyunsaturated, are found mainly in plants and fish—think olives, olive oil, nuts, avocados and salmon. Olive oil and canola oil are especially rich in monounsaturates, and sunflower oil and corn oil are packed with polyunsaturates, including omega-6 fats (though you should avoid consuming too many of these—see page 105).

Many studies have shown that monounsaturated fats in particular can boost the health of your heart. For example, researchers at the University of Pennsylvania found that a diet high in "monos" was twice as effective as a typical low-fat diet at reducing the risk for cardiovascular disease.

That is good news for food lovers. Try cutting down on butter (full of saturated fat) and replace it with olive oil drizzled on crusty bread, or toss a crisp green salad in olive oil mixed with balsamic vinegar (made from healthy grapes).

time for an oil change?

Oils with the most monounsaturated fat and the least saturated fat should be your first choice. The chart shows the proportions of different types of fat in oils commonly used for cooking.

TYPE OF OIL

SATURATED FAT ■ MONOUNSATURATED FAT ■ POLYUNSATURATED FAT ■

canola
safflower
sunflower
corn
peanut
olive
soybean

0g 5g 10g 15g 20g 25g 30g

fat content per 2 tbsp

Omega-3s found in oily fish such as herring help to prevent blood platelets from clumping together and causing heart-stopping blood clots.

and omega-3s

The other form of "good" fats that help to maintain a healthy cardiovascular system are omega-3 fatty acids, also known as essential fatty acids or EFAs. Although they are essential for many body functions, we can't make them in our own bodies, so we must consume them as food.

Omega-3s are found in oily fish such as salmon, fresh tuna, sardines, herring, trout, mackerel and swordfish. They are also present in nuts, leafy green vegetables and a few vegetable oils, such as canola or flaxseed.

Studies indicate that omega-3s help to prevent blood platelets from clumping together and causing heart-stopping blood clots. In the same way, they also lower the risk of strokes caused by clots. They reduce inflammation, high blood pressure and triglyceride levels (see page 101). And there are signs that a diet rich in fish oils blocks the buildup of LDL cholesterol in the aorta, the main artery leaving the heart.

OMEGA-3 vs OMEGA-6

Omega-6 fats, found mostly in processed vegetable oils, are polyunsaturated but should be consumed in limited quantities. It has been demonstrated that very high levels of omega-6 fats in the body can offset the beneficial effects of omega-3s on the cardiovascular system.

The ideal ratio of omega-3s to omega-6 fats is reckoned to be 1:1. But the modern diet tends to include a far higher proportion of omega-6 fats than used to be the case, since they are present in popular cooking oils such as sunflower, safflower and corn oils as well as other processed foods. These days, the typical ratio may be 1:12 or even higher. This imbalance is thought to play a role in the development of inflammation which encourages the formation of plaque in the arteries, one of the characteristics of cardiovascular disease.

eat to beat ...

Your food choices really can help you to live longer. In one study of nearly 4,000 older people, eating oily fish at least once a week was linked with a 44 percent lower risk of dying from a heart attack. Other research shows that omega-3s offer increased protection against a second heart attack.

In one Spanish study, 40 men on a cardiac rehabilitation program were split into two groups. One consumed a dairy product supplemented with omega-3s and vitamins A and D; the other consumed milk with only vitamins A and D. Both groups also underwent a program of supervised exercise. Over the following year, blood homocysteine, a marker of cardiovascular risk, decreased in both groups, but the omega-3 group also had reductions in other cardiovascular disease markers and blood cholesterol levels.

FEAST ON FISH

Eating just two servings of oily fish a week can reduce your risk of heart disease by a third or more. And because of the significant benefits of omega-3s, people who have had a heart attack are recommended to increase their intake to two to four portions weekly. (But it is advisable to eat no more than one portion a week of swordfish, shark or marlin, as they can contain high levels of mercury. Pregnant women or those trying to conceive should avoid them altogether.) To get the maximum benefit from omega-3s, poach, steam, bake or grill your oily fish, rather than frying it.

good fats in fish

Oily fish are better sources of omega-3 fatty acids than white fish. Here are some popular types of fish rated according to their quality as a source of omega-3s.

GREAT SOURCES	MODERATE SOURCES	POOR SOURCES
mackerel	bass	cod
salmon (canned and fresh)	halibut	flounder
sardines	smoked salmon	haddock
sturgeon	sea bass	snapper
trout		sole
tuna (fresh)		tuna (canned)

If you don't like eating fish, consider taking 1 g of fish oil supplement daily. In one four-and-a-half-year Japanese study of over 18,000 people, adding fish oil to cholesterol-lowering statin drug therapy after a heart attack reduced the risk of further major coronary events by around 20 percent.

secret ingredients

Certain important nutrients such as folate and isoflavones have a significant role to play in preventing strokes and heart attacks.

FOLATE

A high level of the protein homocysteine in the blood has been linked with increased rates of cardiovascular disease. For the body to metabolise homocysteine, it needs to take in folate, a B vitamin present in raw fruit and vegetables. Homocysteine and folate levels tend to move in opposite directions. The level of homocysteine increases in people with high blood pressure, but is lowered in response to a good dietary intake of folate and other vitamins.

KEY SOURCES: Peas, broccoli, brussels sprouts, asparagus, chickpeas, brown rice, oranges and bananas.

The level of homocysteine increases in people with high blood pressure, but is lowered in response to a good dietary intake of folate.

ISOFLAVONES

A group of plant chemicals called phytoestrogens mimics some of the effects in the body of the female hormone estrogen—the hormone that, up until menopause, underlies a woman's protection against heart disease. Chief among these phytoestrogens are isoflavones, found particularly in soy and chickpeas.

Dietary isoflavones have been shown to reduce inflammation and stop damaging cells being drawn into arterial plaque. People who include plenty of soy in their diet have lower blood pressure and lower cholesterol levels than those who don't; they are also less likely to become obese, and seem to have more protection against heart attacks and strokes. Isoflavones may help someone avoid a second stroke.

Continued on p. 110 ➤

Mediterranean magic

For many hundreds of years, the people of southern Europe have enjoyed a colorful and delicious diet that has now been shown to provide some protection against heart disease, diabetes and strokes.

FRESH LOCAL CUISINE

The so-called Mediterranean diet—steeped in the culinary traditions of the region, especially southern Italy and Greece—is one of the healthiest diets in the world. As well as being rich in locally grown foods such as olives, olive oil, fresh fruit and vegetables, whole grains and beans, it gives more prominence to freshly caught fish than to red meat.

Even though people in the southern Mediterranean consume relatively high levels of fat, they have far lower rates of cardiovascular disease than North Americans. The type of fats widely eaten in the region actively protect against heart disease by lowering cholesterol, blood pressure and blood sugar. Here, by comparison, we tend to favor polyunsaturated cooking oils such as corn oil, which contains omega-6 rather than omega-3 fats (see page 105), and foods heavy in saturated fat.

THE POWER OF PRODUCE

A key element of the Mediterranean diet is an abundance of fresh fruit and vegetables, which research shows does wonders for cardiovascular health. In one study, scientists measured the vitamin C intake of more than 20,000 men and women, then followed their progress. Nine years later, the people who were consuming higher levels of vitamin C had a 42 percent lower risk of having a stroke. In another study, researchers followed the health of 832 men over a period of 20 years. After analyzing the data and adjusting for age, they found that, on average, each additional three servings of fruit and vegetables a man ate a day lowered his risk of a stroke by more than a fifth. Fruit and vegetables contain a number of vitamins and minerals—such as beta carotene, vitamin C and vitamin E, known as

SECRET weapon

NUTS

If you eat just a small handful of (unsalted) nuts every day for a year—in combination with a Mediterranean diet rich in fruit, vegetables and fish—you are far less likely to die of heart disease or diabetes than people who rarely eat nuts.

Nuts, especially walnuts and pecans, are packed with beneficial omega-3 fatty acids. Walnuts are also rich in vitamin B_6, which helps to control homocysteine, and they provide the amino acid arginine, which stimulates production of nitric oxide, a molecule that relaxes constricted blood vessels. Some research indicates that eating a handful of walnuts just four or five times a week can lower your risk of heart attack by up to 40 percent. Nuts can help to control blood sugar, too. Hazelnuts and cashews contain copper, a nutrient vital for people with diabetes. Harvard scientists found that women who regularly eat a few nuts—any nuts—several times a week are less likely to develop Type 2 diabetes than those who don't.

menu magic

Pick a dish, almost any dish, and add a few nuts to it – for taste and added nutrients. Here are a few simple ideas for incorporating nuts into everyday meals.

- Stir chopped walnuts or pecans into rice dishes.
- Add pistachios to chicken salad.
- Sprinkle your favorite chopped nuts and some dried cranberries on green salads.
- Mix pine nuts or chopped walnuts into pasta dishes along with olive oil, basil and some chopped sun-dried tomatoes.
- Create your own snack mixture with dried fruit, high-fiber cereal and some of your favorite nuts.

antioxidants, which protect the body's cells from harmful free radicals. Fruit and vegetables also add soluble and insoluble fiber to our diet, helping to lower blood cholesterol. That is one reason why medical experts recommend that everyone should eat at least five portions a day—a total of at least 14 oz (400 g). And the more, the better: A 2006 analysis of several different studies found that eating more than five servings a day lowered the risk of stroke by 26 percent.

Oranges are rich in vitamin C—an antioxidant that helps to protect against cardiovascular disease.

WHAT IS A PORTION?

A portion of fruit is any medium-sized piece of fresh fruit, such as an orange, banana or apple; a medium-sized serving of salad or vegetables; or 1/2 cup (125 mL) of stewed or canned fruit. A 1/2 cup (125 mL) of fruit juice also counts, but provides much less useful fiber. If you make just one change to your diet after reading this step, let it be to include fruit and vegetables in every meal you eat. We are lucky to have such a wide variety to choose from— a distinct benefit of the global market, which makes so many countries' produce available to us all year round.

THE GOOD LIFE

A further element of the Mediterranean lifestyle is a love of good red wine, savoured over a leisurely home-prepared family meal that can last for a couple of hours. See page 111 to learn how red wine can help to protect you against cardiovascular disease.

Researchers from the University of Hong Kong studied 102 patients with well-established cardiovascular disease who had experienced a stroke caused by a blood clot in the previous six months. Half the patients received a daily supplement of 80 mg of isoflavones, and the other half were given a placebo. After 12 weeks, there had been a significant improvement in arterial widening among those patients taking isoflavones. The fact that the patients in this trial had relatively advanced cardiovascular disease and had already sustained either a first or second stroke makes the results even more impressive. The greatest benefit was seen among those with the most severe disability. Further research is planned, but the results suggest that eating more isoflavone-rich foods could help to reduce cardiovascular risk in stroke patients—even at a late stage.

KEY SOURCES: Soy, chickpeas, beans, peanuts and green tea.

POLYPHENOLS

Many fruits and vegetables contain antioxidants—chemicals that reduce the level of free radicals in the blood. Free radicals are unstable molecules which, if left to accumulate, cause cell damage. A key group of antioxidants is known as polyphenols, or flavonoids. They reduce inflammation and blood clots, improve the health of arterial linings and lessen other cardiovascular risk factors. In one study of 805 older men, those who consumed the most polyphenols had a 68 percent lower risk of developing cardiovascular disease than those consuming the least.

KEY SOURCES: Berries, apples, beans, peas, cherries, pomegranates, grapes, broccoli, cabbage, onion, sweet potatoes, celery, red wine, green tea, olive oil and chocolate.

calling **chocoholics**

Chocolate-lovers will be delighted to hear that dark chocolate provides protection against heart attacks and strokes. Thanks to its high content of polyphenols and other antioxidants, dark chocolate reduces inflammation, lowers blood pressure, reduces "bad" LDL cholesterol, boosts "good" HDL cholesterol and protects the health of your arteries. It also contains

power foods for healthy arteries

While eating more fruit and vegetables should be high on your list of priorities for boosting the health of your heart and arteries, there are other elements of your diet that can offer significant protection against cardiovascular disease:

● **Red wine**—A polyphenol called resveratrol is thought to be the main ingredient in red wine responsible for its well-documented effect in protecting against heart attacks. British researchers have found that other heart-protecting chemicals, called procyanidins, are especially high in red wines from Sardinia and southwest France.

● **Garlic**—A review of ten studies looking at the effects of garlic on blood pressure showed that, among patients with high blood pressure, garlic supplements produced an average reduction of 16.3 mmHg in systolic and 9.3 mmHg in diastolic blood pressure, compared with patients taking placebo tablets. However, neither had any effect in patients with normal blood pressure.

● **Grapeseed extract**—According to a study involving 24 patients with metabolic syndrome, taking grapeseed extract can lower blood pressure by an average of 12 mmHg systolic and 9 mmHg diastolic after just one month. Participants taking the extract also had reduced LDL cholesterol levels.

> Both green and black tea have been shown to offer protection against cardiovascular disease.

● **Tea**—Both green and black tea have been shown to offer some protection against cardiovascular disease. In one study of 1,900 people taken to the hospital after a heart attack, moderate and heavy tea drinkers had a 31 and 39 percent reduction in the risk of a further event compared with those who hardly drank any tea. However, you may need to take your tea black—according to a study published in the *European Heart Journal*, the protective effects of tea are negated if you add milk.

● **Broccoli** – A diet rich in vegetables from the brassica family, such as broccoli, is known to reduce the risk of heart attacks and strokes. Now scientists from the University of Warwick in the UK have shown that a key broccoli nutrient called sulforaphane can reverse the damage to coronary arteries caused by high blood sugar levels in people with diabetes.

● **Cocoa**—Dutch research reveals that cocoa can lower blood pressure and reduce deaths from cardiovascular disease.

● **Persimmons**—Also called Sharon fruit, persimmons look a little like orange tomatoes. According to research in Israel, they contain a magic cocktail of atherosclerosis-busting chemicals including minerals, antioxidants and trace elements, as well as high levels of dietary fiber. In fact, the researchers recommended a persimmon a day—instead of an apple—to keep the doctor away. There is also evidence from animal research that persimmons improve the metabolism of fats. But if you have had ulcer surgery, avoid the fruit, especially unpeeled; very rarely, they can cause intestinal blockages in people with insufficient stomach acid to digest them properly.

Dean Tarleton

A new attitude to food

When Dean Tarleton suffered a hemorrhagic stroke in March 2007, it left his left arm and leg partially paralyzed. That he had also lost his sense of taste might have seemed a minor problem - except that Dean, then 43, was a chef, running a restaurant at the busy hotel he also owned.

Dean's stroke happened in the early hours as he lay in bed. He remembers trying to get up and just falling to the floor. "It felt as though my arm was made of foam," he says. "My speech had gone and I was gibbering like an idiot." His wife, Vivienne, immediately called an ambulance.

Within 30 minutes Dean was treated in a regional stroke unit. He regained his speech but the weakness down his left side meant he could no longer cook; instead, he supervised the menus.

**"Then, after six months, my taste came back,"
he recalls. "It was wonderful. I really appreciated
the flavors."**

"Then, after six months, my taste came back," he recalls. "It was wonderful. I really appreciated the flavors."

By then, his approach to food had changed - and not just his own food, but his customers', too. High-cholesterol dishes such as creamy peppercorn steaks, deep-fried chicken and fried fish came off the menu, to be replaced with dishes such as grilled fish and steamed vegetables, mostly sourced locally so they were at their peak of freshness. "North Carolina shrimp became very popular," he says.

Dean also benefited personally from adopting a healthier diet, losing 63 lbs, reducing his total cholesterol from 309 to 116 mg/dL (8.0 to 3.0 mmol/L) and lowering his blood pressure.

"I've really embraced the flavors of good food, and realised the benefits of losing weight," Dean says. He advises moderation and wants to spread the healthy-eating message.

"So many things implode in your life after a stroke: Like losing the ability to drive, or small irritations like being unable to reach the end of your belt when it's behind your back." But one good thing has come out of it: "It has really helped me to rediscover the excitement of food."

chemicals that prompt the release of endorphins, the body's pain-relieving and pleasure-promoting hormones. As you will find out in Step 9, a sense of well-being is vitally important to keeping your cardiovascular system in top condition.

In one major review of 139 studies conducted over nearly 40 years, researchers concluded that chocolate consumption could lower the risk of cardiovascular death by around 19 percent. That's the good news. The bad news (for chocoholics) is that all you need to eat to improve your health is 6.7 g per day. That's equivalent to one small square two or three times a week—the heart benefits tend to disappear with consumption of larger amounts. A little dark chocolate may even help to curb our appetite for unhealthier foods, according to research at the University of Copenhagen, which reveals that dark chocolate is more filling

SECRETweapon

CHICKEN SOUP

Researchers in Japan have shown that chicken legs and chicken breast contain chemicals that act like blood pressure-lowering drugs called ACE inhibitors. Early tests were on animals but in February 2009, they published the first human study. Fifteen patients with slightly raised blood pressure took a small daily dose of chicken soup ingredients over four weeks, and their systolic blood pressure (the top figure in a blood pressure reading) dropped by an average 11.8 mmHg.

Eating chocolate could lower the risk of death from cardiovascular disease by around 19 percent.

than milk chocolate and reduces cravings for salty, fatty or sugary items.

The key to eating chocolate is to know when to stop and when not to indulge. A craving for chocolate is the most common of all food cravings in both men and women. If you're hankering for some, try taking a brisk 15-minute walk. Researchers found that a walk allayed cravings in chocoholics, even in tempting situations.

drink to your health

It is now widely accepted that regular, moderate alcohol consumption, especially wine-drinking, is not only enjoyable but can also reduce your risk of coronary artery disease. According to researchers at Joseph Fourier University in France, wine also lowers the risk of second or further heart attacks.

*Indulge in a glass of red wine and savor
a little dark chocolate, knowing that they are
doing you good. Your weight should stay stable.*

When the team studied 353 men who had recently suffered a heart attack, they found that drinking two or more glasses of wine regularly halved their risk of a second attack, compared with men who did not drink.

The benefits of red wine, in particular, are so impressive that at least one British hospital even offers two glasses a day to select heart patients. The key ingredient seems to be a powerful antioxidant called resveratrol, derived especially from Pinot Noir grapes grown in wet and humid regions. If you don't drink, resveratrol can also be found in smaller amounts in grape juice and peanuts. Scientists at the Pavese Pharma Biochemical Institute in Italy are even trying to capture its benefits in a pill.

THE ADVANTAGES OF MODERATION

In the course of a major health study, researchers made some surprising findings about alcohol consumption. They recorded the average weekly alcohol intake of 9,655 civil servants, then logged what happened to them over the following 17 years.

The study concluded that among the group classified at the outset as exhibiting "unhealthy behaviors"—those who smoked, got little or no exercise or had poor dietary habits—moderate drinking was associated with a significant reduction in both fatal and non-fatal heart attacks, compared with abstinence or heavy drinking. In this research, there was no additional benefit derived from alcohol among those initially categorised as exhibiting "healthy behaviors," who did 3 hours or more of exercise per week, ate fruit or vegetables daily and didn't smoke.

healthy weight healthy heart

When it comes to cardiovascular health, the messages are clear: Eat as much natural food—vegetables, fruits and whole grains—as possible; enjoy oily fish such as salmon; and choose olive or canola oil whenever you can. Indulge in a glass of red wine and savor a little dark chocolate, knowing that they are doing you good. Your weight should stay stable. But read on if you are already a little more overweight than is healthy. The same dietary principles apply, but Step 6 explains how you can reduce your calorie intake and shed the excess pounds.

the polymeal

The idea of a polypill that could cure all ills—or, at least, reduce the risk of cardiovascular disease in the majority of the population—was described in Step 1 (see page 34). Well, instead of popping a pill, how about indulging in a delicious meal? That's the proposal made by a team of researchers from the Netherlands, Belgium and Australia. Writing in the *British Medical Journal*, they suggest that their "polymeal" is a more natural, safer and probably tastier alternative to the polypill, and that it could reduce the incidence of cardiovascular disease by as much as 76 percent.

The scientists took published scientific papers that assessed the cardiovascular protective effects of various food ingredients, and came up with an "evidence-based recipe" employing the most efficacious ingredients. Then, using data from major studies of heart disease, they worked out a model of the potential benefits of the polymeal in men and women over the age of 50.

The meal was based on seven food ingredients or categories for which scientific evidence showed specific individual effects in either reducing the incidence of heart attacks and strokes, or in reducing cardiovascular risk factors. These included red wine, fish, dark chocolate, fruit, vegetables, garlic and almonds. Here are the specific calculated effects of each of these ingredients:

- 5 oz (150 mL) red wine daily—reduces cardiovascular disease by 32 percent (though it is advisable to have at least one alcohol-free day a week).
- 4 oz (114 g) fish four times a week—reduces cardiovascular disease by 14 percent.
- 3 ½ oz (100 g) dark chocolate daily—reduces systolic blood pressure by 5.1mmHg and diastolic blood pressure by 1.8 mmHg, equivalent to reducing heart attacks and strokes by 21 percent. (However, as little as 1/3 oz/6.7 g a day is effective, which is worth bearing in mind if you don't want to gain weight.)
- 14 oz (400 g) fruit and vegetables daily—gives the same effect as 3 ½ oz dark chocolate.
- 600 to 900 mg of dried garlic powder a day, or 1–2 cloves of fresh garlic—reduces cholesterol by an amount equivalent to a 25-percent reduction in heart attacks and strokes.
- 2 ½ oz (68 g) almonds daily—reduces total cholesterol by half the amount seen with garlic, equivalent to a reduction in cardiovascular disease of 12.5 percent.

A diet that combined all these ingredients would give a 76 percent reduction in the risk of cardiovascular events in later life, the team calculated. For men, sticking to the polymeal principles after the age of 50 could increase total life expectancy by 6.6 years and yield an extra nine years free of cardiovascular disease. For women, it could add 8.1 years free of cardiovascular disease, and 4.8 years to their total lifespan.

Eating garlic can help to lower cholesterol.

self-defense plan

STEP 6

LOSING EVEN A FEW EXTRA POUNDS CAN MAKE AN ENORMOUS DIFFERENCE TO YOUR HEALTH AND WELL-BEING. YOU'LL NOT ONLY LOOK YOUNGER, YOU'LL FEEL REENERGIZED—AND YOU'LL HAVE THE WONDERFUL SATISFACTION OF KNOWING THAT YOUR WILLPOWER HAS PROBABLY ADDED YEARS TO YOUR LIFE.

Reach your target weight

Do you think you might be too heavy? You're not alone. According to official figures, more than half of us are overweight and one in four is obese. The reasons for this modern affliction are simple: We tend to eat too much of the wrong types of food, and many of us have inactive lifestyles – which means that we are consuming far more calories than our bodies need.

SMART FOOD CHOICES

Step 6 explains how to counter the imbalance between calorie intake and energy expended, and how to compensate for the sedentary working life that is now all too common. As already explained, the types of food that you consume have a huge effect on your weight and the health of your arteries. Simply by making healthier food choices, you will be able to lower your cholesterol and blood pressure and reduce your risk of heart attacks and strokes, as well as that of diabetes, osteoarthritis, liver disease and several forms of cancer. You'll learn, too, why carrying too much fat in certain parts of your body is more dangerous than in others—and when you should worry about the possible health effects.

SECRET OF SUCCESS

Losing weight doesn't have to be a form of punishment. There's no need to spend your days counting

MYTHS X

I WOULD KNOW IF I NEEDED TO LOSE WEIGHT

This is not necessarily the case. More than a quarter of individuals who would be classed by doctors as overweight or obese don't realise that they have a weight problem, according to research carried out by University College London in the United Kingdom. In a survey of 4,000 men and women, in which more than half of the participants were overweight or obese, 87 percent of the obese and 32 percent of the overweight people failed to recognize how heavy they were. Many believed they were a normal weight.

carbohydrates, fat grams and calories. By applying the lessons you learned in Step 5—which foods to eat more of and which to cut back on— you'll make the changes that will ensure you are still trim and healthy ten years from now.

recognize your risk

If you already know you're overweight, it is helpful to know just how heavy you are, so that you can follow your progress as you begin to lose weight. The most reliable indicator of how much body fat you have is the body mass index, or BMI. As explained in Step 3 (see page 66), you can calculate your BMI by multiplying your weight in pounds by 703, and dividing that by your height in inches squared. Look at the information below to find out which weight category you fall into. If you are overweight, it means that you weigh more than the ideal for your sex, height and build; usually, men who are 20 percent or more over their ideal weight, and women who are 25 percent or more over theirs, are obese.

WHAT THE RESULTS MEAN

● A BMI between 18.5 and 24.9 is healthy. For example, the maximum healthy weight of someone who is 5ft 7in tall—male or female—would be around 154 lb.

● If your BMI is between 25 and 29.9, you are officially overweight— meaning you weigh more than you should do based on your age, sex and height. You are more likely to have high blood pressure and are at moderate risk of cardiovascular disease.

● If your BMI is over 30, you are clinically obese and storing far too much fat. You have a high risk of coronary artery disease, high blood pressure, diabetes, heart attacks and strokes.

● A BMI of 40 or more is classed as very or "morbidly" obese, signaling a very high risk of cardiovascular disease and other complications.

If you are overweight or obese according to the height–weight chart, with a BMI of 25 or more, a waist measurement of more than 32 in (80 cm) if you're female or 37 in (94 cm) if you're male, or a waist-to-hip ratio above 0.80 (women) or 0.90 (men), you will experience clear health benefits by losing weight. If you are on the obese side, it is worth talking to your doctor to see if you can get help to do this (see page 122).

Both my parents struggled with obesity. What's the best way for me to avoid getting fat?

People with an obese parent are more likely to be obese themselves. Scientists don't know how much of this is due to genetic inheritance, and how much is due to bad eating habits learned as a child. They do know that we can inherit a tendency to overeat, possibly caused by faulty appetite-control mechanisms that affect the signals which our brains use to detect when we're full. It is not inevitable that people with this tendency will become obese, though they may struggle more than most to control their weight. It is important to be vigilant about diet—about what, and how much you eat—and to build exercise into your daily routine to help to burn off any extra calories.

FIND YOUR MOTIVATION

There are no quick fixes for achieving long-term weight loss. In order to succeed, you must really want to change your eating habits and believe that change is worth the effort. Think about your reasons for wanting to lose weight. You are far more likely to reach your goal if you are pursuing it for your own satisfaction (rather than to appeal to your partner, or to impress your boss, or to stop your neighbor thinking you're fat).

Try to find some inner motivation—such as being able to climb a flight of stairs without panting. Visualize yourself at your ideal weight, feeling attractive, in favorite clothes you haven't been able to wear for a few years—and having the energy and confidence to go swimming with your children. You know what's important to you.

inside information
is obesity caused by a virus?

Could there be a virus that causes obesity? The idea may seem far-fetched, but a nutritional biochemist at Wayne State University in Detroit thinks he has identified just such an organism. In laboratory tests, human adenovirus or AD-36, which is responsible for some cases of respiratory infection, has been shown to cause dramatic weight gain in animals. In an analysis of 1,000 people, another biochemist, Nikhil Dhurandhar, found that those with AD-36 antibodies—a sign that they have been infected with the virus—are significantly more likely to be overweight.

How could a virus make you fat? When fat cells are exposed to AD-36, they begin to multiply, Dhurandhar found. "I'm not saying all obesity is caused by a virus," he says. "Genes, metabolism, habits, all play a role. But at least one other possibility appears to be infection." Scientists are now suggesting that "infectobesity" is worth further investigation.

living life **to the fullest**

For many of us, the most powerful motivation for losing weight is the prospect of feeling fit again, and of being able to live a fuller life. In fact, a landmark study by British researchers clearly indicates that if you lose weight, you will live longer. The scientists analysed BMI data relating to a million people worldwide, who were then followed for up to 20 years. The results show that if you have a BMI of 30 to 35, which is now common, you shorten your life by three years; the seriously obese, with a BMI of 40 to 50, will die ten years earlier than they should. "If you are becoming overweight or obese, avoiding further weight gain could well add years to your life," says epidemiologist Dr. Gary Whitlock of Oxford University, who conducted the study.

TARGET ABDOMINAL FAT

Abdominal fat is especially dangerous because it releases "messenger substances" that promote the development of chronic diseases. It is also linked with metabolic syndrome (see page 30) and the inflammation that provokes the formation of plaque in arteries. Abdominal fat puts you at risk of heart disease, diabetes, high blood pressure and some cancers— even if your overall weight is normal. In a ten-year study involving about 350,000 people, scientists from Imperial College London and the German Institute of Human Nutrition found that a waist measurement of over 39 in (100 cm) in women or 47 in (120 cm) in men more than doubled the risk of premature death, compared to people with a healthy waist size. Other research has found that men and women with high waist-to-hip ratios are almost twice as likely to have calcium deposits inside their coronary arteries—one of the early signs of atherosclerosis.

inside information
the hunger "switch"

Scientists at Canada's Lawson Health Research Institute in London, Ontario have found that abdominal fat releases a hormone called neuropeptide Y, or NPY, that makes more fat cells. High levels of the same hormone in the brain are known to produce constant feelings of hunger and stimulate appetite. If NPY is transported in the blood (the next phase of research will establish whether it is), it may be possible to develop a simple blood test to detect increased levels of NPY in people at risk, and to develop a treatment to "turn off" the hormone.

foods that fight
"middle-age spread"

Abdominal fat is notoriously difficult to get rid of, but here are four foods to include in your healthy diet that will help you to achieve a flatter stomach.

● **Olive oil** Foods that are rich in monounsaturated fat, such as olive oil, contain anti-inflammatory phytochemicals that can help to curb the buildup of abdominal fat. In a 2004 study, 180 people with metabolic syndrome were divided into two groups: 90 followed a Mediterranean diet, rich in olive oil, whole grains, fruits, vegetables and nuts, and 90 followed a relatively high carbohydrate, low-fat diet. Two years later, more than half the dieters in the first group no longer had metabolic syndrome—they had lost weight and had healthier cholesterol levels. Inflammation in their arteries dropped dramatically, and tests indicated that the lining of their blood vessels was much healthier too. They also showed less evidence of insulin resistance, which increases the risk for Type 2 diabetes and heart disease. In the control group which didn't follow the diet, 78 of 90 participants still had metabolic syndrome.

Green tea stimulates fat-burning in the body and abdominal fat in particular.

● **Nuts** Eating a small handful of nuts every day could help to reverse metabolic syndrome. That's the implication of a Spanish study, in which participants who ate a Mediterranean diet—along with extra nuts—for a year reduced their abdominal fat, blood pressure and cholesterol levels. Nuts contain anti-inflammatory substances such as fibre and antioxidants such as vitamin E. **A note of caution:** Adding nuts, which are high in calories, to a diet already packed with too many calories and junk food could lead to weight gain.

● **Soy protein** In one small study, women who drank a soy-based drink daily gained less abdominal weight than those who drank a milkshake. The researchers speculate that it is the isoflavones in soy that protect against adding fat in this area. Try edamame (fresh green soy beans, available shelled or in the pod), soy nuts, tofu, miso soup and soy milk.

● **Green tea** In one study, volunteers were given a daily drink of green tea, which contains catechins, an antioxidant. (The daily dose was 625 mg; an average cup of green tea has from 150 to 250 mg.) After 12 weeks, the group had a significant reduction in abdominal fat and triglycerides. Green tea may also increase the body's sensitivity to insulin, lowering the risk of diabetes.

If you've tried to lose weight but just can't make any progress, talk to your doctor.

How your **doctor can help**

The brutal truth is, sometimes the enemy has simply gained too much ground. For many people who have high blood pressure, diabetes, metabolic sydrome, angina, or who have had a stroke or heart attack, losing weight is particularly hard. If you've tried to lose weight but just can't make any progress, talk to your doctor. He or she will be used to giving advice about this problem, and will probably be delighted that you've decided to tackle it.

Your doctor can discuss lifestyle factors with you and help you to set a target weight and realistic timeframe for achieving it. Some hospitals run obesity clinics. Alternatively, your doctor may refer you to a dietitian or nutritionist for practical dietary advice, or to a weight-loss counseling program.

PILLS ARE NO PANACEA
If you have a high BMI combined with an existing condition such as high blood pressure, high cholesterol or diabetes, your doctor may prescribe medication to aid weight loss. These drugs are not magic pills, however—you will still need to eat well and exercise. They are prescribed only to those who have demonstrated that they can lose weight on a calorie-controlled diet.

Xenical, or orlistat, works by blocking the absorption of some fats in the intestines, and the makers claim that it can boost weight loss by 50 percent compared with dieting alone. You need to take care not to eat too much fat while taking Xenical, or you may suffer side effects such as diarrhea and gas. Orlistat is also available in lower doses in the United States as over-the-counter product Alli. Other prescription-only medications available in the US include phentermine and diethylpropion, which affect appetite.

THE SURGICAL OPTION

If you are extremely obese, with a BMI of 40 or higher, or a BMI of 35 or higher with one or more severe medical conditions related to weight, such as coronary artery disease or diabetes, you may be eligible for something called bariatric surgery, to reduce the size of your stomach.

GASTRIC BANDING

Gastric banding, or gastric restriction, involves placing a band around the upper part of the stomach to restrict the amount you can eat and make you feel full even though you have eaten a relatively small amount. This can be done through laparoscopic surgery techniques, so scarring is minimal. The band includes a fluid-filled balloon connected to an injection port brought out through the skin. It can be adjusted by injecting or withdrawing fluid to tighten or loosen the band as needed. It can also be removed altogether when required, so the procedure is reversible.

GASTRIC BYPASS

The most common bariatric procedure in North America is the gastric bypass method known as "stomach stapling," which physically restricts the amount you can eat by creating a small pouch stapled off from the main part of the stomach. A section of the small intestine is then bypassed and reconnected to the pouch. As a result, all food eaten takes a shorter route through the stomach and less is digested. The procedure is typically performed laparoscopically. This procedure usually leads to more weight loss than gastric banding, and that loss is both faster and more likely to be maintained. Though stomach stapling has a slightly higher complication rate, overall complications rates are relatively low when performed by experienced surgeons. There are other gastric bypass methods as well; discuss the options with your doctor to see which method is best for you.

troubleshooting Q&A

Could my obesity be due to a medical problem?

Medical causes of obesity are fairly uncommon, but if you do have sudden, unexplained weight gain, tell your doctor. It may be due to an underactive thyroid; other symptoms include tiredness, depression, dry skin, constipation, aches and hair loss. If weight gain is accompanied by swollen ankles, it could be a sign of heart failure due to fluid retention. Another disorder characterized by weight gain, which affects 6–8 percent of women of childbearing age, is polycystic ovary syndrome. Some medications such as steroids prescribed for other conditions can cause weight gain.

crash diets don't work

Skip the fad diets. They simply don't work, partly because they are usually too drastic to maintain for the rest of your life. Also, many of these diets lack sufficient scientific research to support their occasionally ridiculous claims.

Also, even though you might seem to lose a lot of weight at the beginning of such diets, most of that weight loss is actually water loss; your body is burning up stored sugars that previously soaked up excess water. Then you reach the "plateau" phase, after which further weight loss is increasingly difficult—that's when most people become discouraged.

One review of 31 studies shows clearly how often deliberate dieting fails in the long term. While the subjects lost weight in the first six months, within five years, two-thirds put on more weight than they had initially lost. In one study, half the dieters were 11 lb heavier than their initial weight.

The truth is that the human body has evolved to survive periods of reduced food intake by going into "starvation mode." This involves adjusting its metabolism—the rate at which it burns calories—to try to conserve energy. So, if you drastically reduce your calorie intake, your body will react by starting to burn fewer calories to keep your body's normal processes functioning. It learns to

SECRET weapon

21ST-CENTURY FOOD DIARY

Watching what you eat has taken on a new meaning in the digital age. People who are trying to lose weight should photograph their food before eating it, suggest American scientists who compared the usefulness of ordinary written food diaries with photographic diaries.

The researchers found that, when volunteers took a snapshot of each meal before they ate it, they were more conscious of what they were about to eat, were frequently prompted to eat more healthily and were less likely to overeat. Photographs are accurate, simple and quick, and may act as a brake on bingeing, the researchers say. You don't even need a camera; use your cell phone if that's easiest. These snapshots could make you stop and think before you chow down.

Photograph your food—these snapshots could make you stop and think before you chow down.

ten weight-loss winners

The key to successful weight loss involves making small but important changes that you can incorporate easily into your everyday routine. After tracking a group of volunteers over eight weeks and monitoring their behaviour relating to food and eating, researchers came up with these ten tips that have proven to be effective:

1 Keep to your meal routine Whether you have two, three, four or five daily meals, try to eat them at roughly the same times each day.

2 Reduce fat Choose reduced-fat versions of foods such as dairy products, spreads and salad dressings where you can. Use sparingly and check the labels carefully; although the fat level has been "reduced," some may still be relatively high in fat.

3 Walk off the weight Walk 10,000 steps (equivalent to 60–90 minutes of moderate activity) each day. You can use a pedometer to count the steps and spread the exercise through the day.

4 Pack a healthy snack If you like to eat snacks, choose a healthy item such as a piece of fresh fruit or low-calorie yogurt, instead of chocolate or chips.

5 Look at the labels Be careful about food claims. Check the fat and sugar content on food labels when shopping and preparing food.

6 Careful with your portions Don't heap food (except vegetables) onto your plate. Think twice before having second helpings.

7 Get up on your feet Break up the time you spend sitting. Stand up for 10 minutes of every hour.

8 Think about your drinks Choose water or unsweetened fruit juice. The latter is high in natural sugar, so try to limit it to one glass per day (8 fl oz/240 mL). Alcohol is high in calories, so try to limit the amount you drink.

9 Focus on your food Slow down. Don't eat while you are walking around or watching television. Eat at a table if possible.

10 Don't forget your veggie servings Eat at least seven (preferably nine or ten) servings of fruit and vegetables a day .

expect a lower food intake. As soon as your calorie intake increases, you are even more likely to gain weight until your body adjusts again—and that could take months, during which time you're piling on the pounds.

FALSE PROMISES

Even worse than one-off crash diets is the phenomenon known as "yo-yo" dieting, or weight cycling, in which people get trapped in a pattern of weight loss followed by weight gain, followed by further dieting to lose weight again. Typically, someone who is overzealous about losing weight quickly picks an extreme diet and—if they can stick to it for a while—is initially overjoyed at the amount of weight lost in a short time. But diets that deprive you of too much are impossible to follow for long, and they make you irritable, tired and depressed. They also intensify food cravings and encourage you to eat too much when you stop the diet. As a result, you feel like a failure—even though it was the fad diet that failed, not you.

THE BIG DANGER

If you lose weight too quickly through crash dieting alone, the big danger is that you will lose muscle mass as well as body fat, particularly if you are not doing exercise. Since muscle burns far more calories than fat, losing muscle mass is bad news.

When you stop dieting and start eating more, you will only gain fat unless you are exercising as well. So what crash dieting does is swap muscle for fat, increasing your fat-to-muscle ratio as well as slowing your metabolism, and causing weight gain in the long term.

Studies show that crash dieting reduces levels of HDL (the "good" cholesterol), slows cardiac blood flow in postmenopausal women and actually increases your proportion of body fat. You are much more likely to lose weight permanently by making small, sustained changes to your eating habits.

ways in which the body uses food

Scientists believe that arginine, an essential amino acid in our bodies, could be a useful weapon in the battle against obesity. Researchers at A&M University in Texas fed obese rats either a high- or a low-fat diet supplemented with arginine for 12 weeks. They found that, by regulating the quantity of the amino acid given to the rats, they were able to increase muscle mass and significantly reduce body fat in both groups—by 63 and 65 percent respectively. The scientists say that arginine alters the way the body uses food. They are planning to do follow-up studies in obese adults and children to test the benefits of taking supplements. Arginine-rich foods include watermelon, seafood, nuts, seeds, algae, meat and soy protein.

And to ensure that you achieve steady gradual weight loss, it is best to combine healthier eating with more exercise. Most overweight or obese people should aim to lose between 5 and 10 percent of their starting weight in the first three months of a weight-loss program. You should soon notice the positive effect on your health, particularly if you are already suffering from high blood pressure, diabetes or arthritis.

Diets that deprive you of too much are impossible to follow for long, and make you irritable, tired and depressed.

your healthy **eating plan**

The key to successful weight loss is to eat healthy foods in moderation. So when you're thinking about adopting a new eating plan, start by taking a long, hard look at your current diet. Review the results of the questionnaires in Step 3, then apply the lessons you learned about "good foods" in Step 5.

Your target is to eat more natural, unprocessed foods and cut down on take-out, instant meals and fried foods that are high in saturated fat, sugar and salt. Choose more fruit, vegetables, fish, lean protein and unsaturated fats. And don't forget whole grains such as whole

> Breakfast reduces cravings for high-fat or sugary snacks later in the day, and increases people's fruit and vegetable intake.

wheat bread, brown rice and cereals that still have their fibre-rich outer layer. The benefit of whole grains lies in the fact that they take a long time for your body to break down; they satisfy your hunger but don't pile on the calories. Try to have three servings every day. These are nutrient-dense rather than calorie-dense foods that provide substantial amounts of vitamins and minerals, and fewer empty calories.

NICE AND SIMPLE

The beauty of the healthy eating plan outlined above is its simplicity. There is no need to spend hours counting carbohydrates, fat grams or calories.

You simply learn which foods to eat more of, and which foods to cut back on. Even the small changes in calorie intake that this will generate will make a difference. Provided that you continue to take in fewer calories than your current level, and that you burn off more energy than you take in as food, you will soon start to shed unwanted pounds.

SUSTAINING WEIGHT LOSS

Once you have made a decision to manage your weight, it is something you need to continue to do for the rest of your life. The plan described in these pages adds up to a life-long strategy, not a short-term (and potentially dangerous) fix. The encouraging news is that these minor adjustments can contribute to significant weight loss over time. Depending on the quality of your diet at the moment, you may find that just following the good-diet guidelines in Step 5 will help you to take off the pounds gained over years of less healthy eating.

A NOTE ABOUT CALORIES

When referring to energy intake and expenditure, we usually talk about "calories," but we're actually talking about kilocalories, or Cal (also known as the "large" or "food" calorie). This may seem confusing, but it's because a calorie, in strict scientific terms, is a tiny unit of heat energy equal to that needed to heat 1 gram's worth of water by 1°C. So it's easier to measure in food calories, each of which is equal to 1,000 small calories.

inside information
men may be able to "switch off"

Men may find it easier than women to avoid tempting food when they are on a diet and could even find it easier to lose weight. In a brain-scan study, researchers flashed tempting foods in front of men and women who hadn't eaten for a day, then told them to fight their hunger. The men's brains showed far less activity in areas of emotional regulation, memory and motivation than the women's—as if men were more easily able to "switch off" their cravings for favorite foods, which included fried chicken, lasagna, ice cream and pizza.

Whether you are male or female, however, your willpower can be undermined by stress and anxiety. So if you are trying to lose weight and you have just had a difficult day at the office, don't walk home past a bakery.

golden rules

During the first weeks of adjusting to a healthy eating plan, your willpower will probably be pushed to the limit. Described below are some golden rules to help keep you on track.

One very useful tactic is to keep a food diary. For the first week, make a record of every item of food and drink that you consume, at what time and how you feel (or take pictures—see page 124). The diary will enable you to review your choices and take stock of what prompts you to eat. You need to learn how to distinguish between true biological hunger— the sign of a healthy appetite—and false alarms, when you feel the urge to eat because you are bored or stressed.

(or take pictures—see page 124)

DEFENSEtactics

PORTION PROPORTIONS

We have become so used to seeing (and eating) big portion sizes that many of us don't recognize what a moderate-sized serving actually looks like.

Here are some examples of moderate servings with illustrative comparisons:

- 3 oz (90 g) of meat **the size of a pack of cards**
- 1 baked potato **a clenched fist**
- 1 1/2 oz (45 g) oatmeal (uncooked) **1/3 of a coffee mug**
- 1 oz (25 g) cheese **four stacked playing dice**
- Butter or margarine on bread/toast **a nickel**
- Nuts or dried fruit **a golf ball**
- Pasta, rice, mashed potato **a computer mouse**
- 6 fl oz (180 mL) juice **a small yogurt container**

(Generally, there is no need to limit portion sizes of fruit and vegetables.)

SCHEDULE SMALLER MEALS

Scheduling breakfast, lunch, dinner and snacks in the same way that you schedule other daily appointments can help to prevent overeating, so take your meals at regular, set times. Eating small amounts, often improves appetite control, reduces hunger and avoids the blood-sugar swings that can induce you to eat more. In one study, men who increased their frequency of eating consumed up to 27 percent fewer calories. Instead of three large meals, try to build five or six small portions of healthy foods into your daily routine.

CHOOSE HEALTHY SNACKS

Whenever you reach for a snack, think about why you are doing it. Because the food's there? Because you feel upset or tired? Eating can be an emotional reaction, and once you understand why you crave a sugary doughnut or cookie, you may find it easier to resist. It's also worth keeping healthy snacks at hand so you can satisfy momentary hunger without upsetting your general diet. Choose snacks that add nutrients and keep you feeling full, such as fruit or cut-up vegetables— keep a stock of chopped carrots and broccoli in the fridge.

sensible snacking

Most of us love to nibble. In fact, we eat an average of three snacks a day. While there is nothing wrong with snacking in itself, all too often we fill ourselves up on high-calorie, high-fat snack foods, then either skimp on meals that contain important nutrients or eat normal-sized meals and consume too many calories in total.

There is a way to snack sensibly, however: Choose nutritious snacks, and think of them as part of your daily food intake rather than as "extras." This will satisfy your cravings and help you to meet your nutritional needs. Instead of potato chips, try a piece of fruit or a container of low-fat yogurt.

SNACK	CAL
9 fl oz (250 mL) tomato juice	35
1 oz (25 g) ready-to-eat dried apricots	40
1 medium apple	47
4 oz (100 g) grapes	60
1 medium banana	95
1 low-fat granola bar	95
1 English muffin with 2 tsp reduced-sugar jam	100
1 slice of whole wheat bread with cottage cheese	100
6 oz (200 g) container low-fat yogurt	125
5 1/4 oz (150 g) low-fat rice pudding	150

AVOID THESE TREATS They may seem light, but they pack a high-calorie punch.

1 small croissant	230
2 chocolate cookies	168
1 small bag potato chips	150
1 small bag cheese puffs	155

EAT SMALLER PORTIONS

Many of us have gotten used to eating far more than we need. One reason is that average portion sizes of restaurant and fast-food meals, pastries and other prepared foods have increased dramatically over the last two decades. Some have nearly doubled in size, even in restaurants. We tend to serve more at home too—portions are now up to eight times as large as those recommended.

Try serving food on smaller plates. This can cut the amount of food eaten by as much as 25 percent, according to psychologists at Cornell University. Other studies reveal that people consume 34 percent fewer liquid calories when they drink out of tall, skinny glasses instead of short, stubby ones.

EASY EATING ADJUSTMENTS

- Cut your portion sizes by around 10 percent. When you get used to the smaller size, reduce portions by another 10 percent.
- Use slightly less butter and slightly less cooking oil. Consider switching to a low-fat margarine.
- If you tend to splurge on snack foods such as cookies, buy individually wrapped items. Having to open each packet in turn will discourage you from overindulging.
- Bake, steam or grill food instead of frying it.
- Have one meal each day that excludes starchy carbohydrates (no rice, potatoes, pasta or bread). Try a lean chicken breast with salad or two portions of different vegetables, for example.
- Trim all visible fat from meat and remove the skin from poultry.
- Replace sugary breakfast cereal with a slice of whole wheat toast and a piece of fruit.
- When eating out in restaurants, choose tomato-based sauces rather than creamy ones.

make every meal a pleasure

As described in Step 5, people who live in the Mediterranean countries of southern Europe eat a very different diet from most people in North America. They eat more healthily and are less likely to gain weight as they get older—two factors that are thought to explain at least some of the variations between countries in the prevalence of heart disease and strokes. But is the content of their diets all that's involved?

Southern Europeans (think Italy, Greece and Spain) generally take more time over their meals and tend to ensure that they eat in pleasant surroundings, at an attractively laid table free of clutter—TV dinners are not part of the agenda. They savor their food, lingering, chatting, making meals into social occasions. This style of dining is beneficial to health in all kinds of ways: Being social is good for your heart, as indicated in Step 9, and it may also hold a clue to losing weight.

Habitually hurrying your meals doubles your risk of being overweight, according to one study of 3,000 people. Why? Eating fast could mean that there's not enough time for your stomach to send "I'm full" signals to your brain to tell you to stop eating before you consume too much. And the simple act of chewing may send other signals that cause your brain to feel satisfied and release appetite-suppressing hormones—but only

A good night's sleep can help you to resist food cravings.

20 minutes or more after you start to eat. Those in the study who both ate fast and continued eating until they felt full were three times as likely to be overweight as those who did neither of these things. So if you wolf down too much too quickly, your body's natural feedback mechanisms are unable to keep up. It appears that some "fast food" may be dangerous because of the speed at which it's generally eaten, as well as because of its contents.

SLOW DOWN

Deliberately trying to savor your food could have other benefits. Several studies suggest that obese people actually derive less pleasure from food than people of normal weight—and that they eat more in an attempt to increase their sense of satisfaction. In reinforcement of this theory, researchers have now shown that some people have a particular genetic makeup that adversely affects the quantity of gratification-promoting chemicals in their brain.

So eat slowly, take time to relish your food, put your knife and fork down at intervals. Never eat lunch at your desk, while talking on the phone or answering emails. If you do, you are more likely to overeat.

SECRETweapon

SLEEP WELL

Getting a good night's sleep can build up your resistance to food cravings. Sleep is crucial in regulating metabolism, so, when you get the seven to eight hours a night most people need, you feel rejuvenated. But just one night of sleep deprivation significantly increases feelings of hunger, and people who are deprived of sleep double their risk of obesity, research finds. Inadequate sleep reduces levels of leptin, the hormone that signals to the body when we are full, while increasing levels of ghrelin, the hormone that makes us feel hungry.

When sleep scientists at the University of Chicago limited healthy volunteers to four hours of sleep a day, their leptin levels were similar to those of people underfed by 1,000 Cal a day for three days. In a similar study, sleep-deprived men and women craved sweets and starchy and salty foods. For advice on what to do about sleep problems, see Step 9.

a winning combination

Reducing the amount you eat or doing more exercise will help you to lose weight, but for maximum effect you need to do both. This approach is also the best way to protect your cardiovascular system.

ENERGY STORAGE

One reason why many of us gain weight in middle age is because we are less physically active as we get older. That tendency is made worse by the fact that we don't have to expend as much energy as we used to, simply to survive—nor, in the days of central heating, do we need fat layers to keep us warm. We have cars and buses and trains to save us from traveling on our own steam, and a vast range of machines and gadgets to save us from effort in everyday life. But humans have evolved to store body fat as a reserve for times of famine, and some people will do this more efficiently than others. An obese person can store up to a year's worth of energy as fat. The problem is that, when food is in plentiful supply, that is just too much to get used up during an ordinary day.

A TWO-PRONGED ATTACK

In one study of obese, inactive men and women with poor glucose tolerance (suggesting a high risk of diabetes), a 12-week program of aerobic exercise reduced body fat without affecting lean muscle mass, and improved both fitness and blood sugar levels—but greater improvements were seen among those who also followed a reduced-calorie diet. In another study, reported in the *International Journal of Obesity*, researchers proved that exercise is vital to reducing the size of abdominal fat cells—calorie restriction alone just didn't work. That's important, because fat-cell size has been shown to predict the risk of diabetes, whether or not someone is actually obese.

REDalert **!**

COUCH POTATOES

The more time you spend watching television, the more likely you are to become obese and to develop diabetes. That's the conclusion of a six-year study involving 50,000 women. Researchers found that an additional two hours watching TV was associated with a 25 percent greater risk of obesity and a 14 percent increased risk of diabetes. What's more, the dangers persisted even when the statistics were adjusted to take account of other factors such as diet and smoking. So it's not just increased snacking while you're watching that's responsible, nor is it simply sitting—the perils of which are discussed in the next chapter. The researchers discovered that risks were also increased when office workers sat for similar periods, but not by nearly as much as television-watching. They recommend limiting your television time to no more than ten hours per week. People in North America currently watch, on average, 21 hours of television a week.

A PLAN FOR ALL AGES

You're never too old to benefit from a health program. Researchers in Taiwan identified 52 younger and 50 older people, all of whom were obese and had diabetes, and put them on a one-year program that combined a calorie-reducing diet and moderate aerobic-exercise regime. At the end of the year, improvements in BMI, total cholesterol and triglycerides were the same in both age groups, while improvements in body-fat levels, waist circumference and various metabolic markers were actually better among the older participants.

SET REALISTIC TARGETS

Avoid setting overambitious targets. The key to success in any weight-loss regime is to make changes that you can easily incorporate into your everyday life. As an example, if you can burn just an extra 58 Cal each day—from 10 minutes of dancing, for example—while keeping the same food intake, you will lose half a pound a month. Take in 58 Cal less food each day as well—the equivalent of one cookie—and you'll double this. That could add up to 12 lb in a year, with hardly any extra effort. Obviously, with a little bit more exertion and a little bit less food, you'll lose even more. Sticking to one element of a plan, whether it's to get more exercise or cut down on junk food, boosts your willpower and self-control, making you more likely to succeed in other areas.

DEFENSEtactics

A MIX OF EXERCISE IS BEST

For the most effective weight loss, make sure that you do both aerobic exercise and strength training. Aerobic exercise—the type that makes you breathe faster and stimulates blood circulation—is ideal for the health of your cardiovascular system. It also speeds up metabolism (the rate at which you burn calories), but only for a short time. Strength training—which builds up muscle mass—helps to boost your metabolism overall, because the muscle mass that you are gaining burns up more calories than the fat that you are shedding. And it's beneficial to incorporate some stretching exercises too, to enhance flexibility and help keep you mobile. See Step 7 for more details.

A two-pronged attack—tackling both diet and exercise—is vital if you're serious about losing weight.

Jackie Herbert

Weight-loss triumph

When Jackie Herbert was diagnosed with diabetes five years ago, at the age of 52, she weighed 225 lb. She'd mentioned to her doctor that she had to get up frequently at night to urinate and was also very thirsty. "He tested my blood sugar and told me I had diabetes. Then he said I needed to lose weight."

Jackie managed to lose more than 28 lb in eight months. "I simply stopped buying fatty foods such as sausage biscuits and cake, and I used only small amounts of oil in cooking," she says. Before eating anything, she'd ask herself, "Should I eat this? Is it fattening?" Slowly the weight began to drop off - and she helped her husband, Eddie, to lose 28 lb too. "It was easier with Eddie's support, but I would have lost weight on my own because I knew this time I had to do something."

Jackie had gained weight after menopause, and thinks her diet was largely to blame. Now she eats more fresh food, and moderation is her motto. "Life is for living. I'm not going to give up everything. If I want some chocolate, I have some, but a small amount - and I make sure it's good quality."

Before eating anything, Jackie would ask herself, "Should I eat this? Is it fattening?'

She also keeps active, looking after her four-year-old grandson four days a week, plus her own cleaning, cooking, washing, ironing and household chores when required. It all helps to keep the weight off, she says.

"I've lost another 7 lb in the last eight weeks," Jackie adds, and thinks this may also be due to a newly acquired taste for Japanese food. "I've been making lots of sushi, which is small in terms of quantity but filling. I also make bread - pounding the dough is pretty good exercise."

Her new lifestyle is paying dividends. While Jackie still needs medication for diabetes and cholesterol-lowering drugs, her cholesterol levels are normal and her blood sugar is down.

"Diabetes is in my life, but I don't let it rule me. It only becomes an issue if you ignore the rules. I take my tablets, watch what I eat and keep my blood sugar under control. But I still live life to the fullest. I won't let it change me."

BUILD UP YOUR ACTIVITY LEVEL

Small daily additions to your activity level can often make more difference than an all-out crash exercise program that you probably won't be able to sustain (and which may be harmful if you do).

It takes 3,500 Cal to make 1 lb of fat, and you need to burn this amount to lose it. Half an hour of brisk walking will burn up about 150 Cal; if you do that five days a week, you'll burn enough calories to lose 11 lb in the course of a year, as long as you don't increase your food intake.

the **neat** solution

We all use energy each day simply to stay alive and keep our bodies in working order. This is known as "basal metabolism." It takes on average, about 1,300 Cal for women and 1,600 Cal for men—that's what we would use up if we did nothing but lie down or sleep all day. For those people who have a fairly inactive lifestyle, basal metabolism may account for as much as 60 percent of their total energy expenditure.

In addition to this, of course, we use up energy and burn calories during physical exertion. According to Dr. James Levine of the Mayo Clinic, we do this in one of two ways: "One is to go to the gym, and the other is through all the activities of daily living called NEAT—Non-Exercise Activity Thermogenesis." (Thermogenesis means heat generation, a product of the breakdown of food to create energy). NEAT is the energy used up in routine daily activities, when we're doing more than just lying down, but not actually "exercising"—washing up the dishes or taking out the garbage, rather than jogging or playing soccer.

For most people in Western societies, NEAT is by far the most significant form of energy expenditure, says Dr. Levine. "In people who have sedentary lifestyles, NEAT is responsible for less than 15 percent of total energy expenditure, whereas it may account for more than 50 percent in highly active people. It appears that NEAT is far more important for calorie-burning than exercise in nearly everyone." A study of 20 volunteers at the Mayo Clinic proves his point.

MYTHS X

SWEAT MORE, LOSE MORE

The common belief that the more profusely you sweat during exercise, the more calories you burn, has no basis in fact. It is true that strenuous exercise burns up more calories than gentle exercise, but sweating is not a reliable indicator of strenuous exercise. What's more, sweating simply sheds water—so any weight lost directly as a result of sweating will be put straight back on when you have a drink afterward.

The results demonstrated that "it's metabolically more effective to put more NEAT into your life to achieve a healthy body weight than to seek organized exercise." Even minor changes in physical activity throughout the day can increase daily energy expenditure by around 20 percent.

ON THE GO

So how do you get more NEAT into your life? The answer is through just about anything involving movement that's not strictly "exercise." Examples include certain aspects of your work, your housework and leisure activities. Even fidgeting counts; according to researchers in the US and Germany, some people have a hereditary "fidget" gene—and inveterate fidgets are less likely to be overweight than others. If you are someone who shuffles and shifts in your seat, fiddles with pencils or

You're on the way to taking control of your weight – rather than letting it control you.

taps your feet, you're getting valuable daily exercise without even knowing it, they say. In a study at the Mayo Clinic, Dr. Levine fed 16 people an extra 1,000 Cal a day. After two months, the natural fidgeters in the group weighed the same; those who barely moved had gained 12 lb. Fidgeting can burn up to 350 Cal a day. Over the course of a year, that's equivalent to working off up to 40 lb of fat.

in the driver's seat

Step 6 has explained why the best way to keep your weight down is to make small changes to your eating patterns and daily activity levels. You don't need to embark on a crash diet or join a gym, but you do need to be patient. Most people who weigh more than is healthy have gained weight gradually over months or years, and it may take some time to lose it. Don't weigh yourself more than once every week or, preferably, every two weeks. There are two reasons for following this advice. First, you may be fooled by an initial improvement that is in fact mostly water loss, then get downhearted when it's not sustained. Second, you may see no change at all, or—if you have just started exercising regularly for the first time—even an early increase, because your new muscle weighs more than fat. Again, this can be discouraging. Keep track of your waist measurement as well as your weight; waist measurements are actually more important. But again, don't measure too often.

And remember that you're most likely to succeed if you adopt realistic goals. The key is small, steady changes of around 1 lb a week, so there's no point weighing yourself more often. Many people find interim goals help their progress; aim to lose 4½ lb by Easter, trim an inch in time for your summer vacation or go down a clothing size in three months.

KEEP IT UP

If you have begun to adopt more careful eating habits, you're already on the way to controlling your weight, rather than letting it control you. Now you have to plan how to keep the weight off in the long term. Many people need as much support to maintain their reduced weight as they did to lose it in the first place. Your chances of success will be boosted—and you'll be far more likely to carry on with your healthy diet—if everyone in the family adopts similar habits, than if you have to shop and cook separate meals for yourself.

Support can come from many sources—not just from your family, but also from friends, your doctor, a weight-loss support group or an exercise class including other people who have the same aim as you.

TIME TO GET MOVING

You know the dangers of being overweight. You have assessed your own risk and can apply what you have learned about different types of food that can help you to fulfill your weight-loss program.

Of course, no plan for losing weight and protecting your heart and arteries is complete without regular exercise. In Step 7 you will discover how to get started on an exercise regime. You will learn some dos (exercise should be enjoyable and fun) and don'ts (if you push yourself too hard and too fast, you are much more likely to give up). And as you embark on a strategy for incorporating more physical activity into your life—so you can both shed pounds and keep them off—you may find it's easier than you think.

self-defense plan
STEP
7

YOU KNOW THAT EXERCISE IS GOOD FOR YOUR HEALTH, BUT THE HARDEST PART IS GETTING STARTED—OR IS IT? AS YOU'LL DISCOVER, YOU DON'T HAVE TO JOIN A GYM OR RUN FOR MILES TO GIVE YOUR ARTERIES A WORKOUT. ALL IT TAKES IS A CONSCIOUS DECISION TO GET UP AND GET MOVING IN EVERYDAY LIFE.

Get in
shape

The word "exercise," with its implications of exhausting gym workouts or five-mile runs, might discourage many people. But you don't have to be a dedicated athlete to maintain the health of your heart and arteries. What counts is keeping as active as you can in your daily life and squeezing a little more physical activity into everything you do. If you adopt this holistic approach, you'll get to watch your energy levels rise as your weight falls.

BREAKING BAD HABITS

As far as our bodies are concerned, 21st-century life can be surprisingly static, and it takes a determined effort to change habits that have become deeply ingrained. In our technologically advanced, automated world, more and more of us spend our days doing sedentary office jobs. Not only that, but thanks to modern appliances, housework is much less arduous than it used to be. So although our days go by at a frantic pace, our lives do not often involve physical challenges; to get around quickly, we rely on cars, and after a stressful, mentally tiring day, many of us choose to relax in front of the television.

Fewer than half of American adults get the recommended amount of moderate exercise five or more days a week, or intense exercise three times a week, which are required to protect the cardiovascular system. And as we get older, we exercise less. A government survey found that just 27 percent of women aged 75 or older and 38 percent of men aged 75 or older met the recommendations. Stats for Canadians aren't much better, prompting experts to decry the inactivity plague in that country, too. It is hard to break free from the vicious cycle: You put on weight, you get less exercise, you put on more weight and so on. This pattern is clearly damaging. One study estimated that as many as one in five medically-related deaths of people over 35 can be partly attributed to a lack of exercise.

EXERCISE IS FUN

The key to changing your own life is to opt for activities you want to do. Go dancing, enroll in a yoga class, kick a soccer ball with your kids, take the stairs instead of the elevator or just walk in the countryside on a glorious summer evening. It's up to you to choose which physical activities you incorporate into your daily routine—and every little bit counts.

Kick a soccer ball with your kids.

powerful health benefits

The benefits of exercise are so stunning that if they could be packaged as a pill, it would be considered a miracle cure. Regular, moderate exercise halves your risk of heart disease and strokes over the long term, and makes you five times less likely to die from cardiovascular disease than someone whose daily routine involves no physical exertion. A Scottish study estimates that reducing levels of inactivity by just 1 percent a year for five years would, in Scotland alone, prevent 2,162 deaths from heart disease and 128 from strokes.

Exercise can even bring benefits to people who already have heart disease. A Norwegian study that was conducted over a period of 18 years clearly indicated that both women and men with coronary disease who exercised for just half an hour a week were likely to live longer than those who did no exercise. The more exercise they did, the greater their longevity.

troubleshooting Q&A

I'm 68. I used to be pretty active but I lost the habit. What kinds of exercise would be best for me?

The best activities for someone in your situation include brisk walking, Pilates and isometric exercises (see pages 160–61), which will all help to prevent the muscle loss that tends to occur with age. Since muscle naturally burns more calories than other tissue, you will also store less fat.

It is never too late to build up your muscle strength. In one study of volunteers in their nineties who followed an eight-week strength-training program, some increased their strength threefold. As you get more active, you will also build up your aerobic capacity (how well your heart and lungs deal with exercise). Just remember to take it in slow, steady stages if you've been inactive for a while.

Exercise that strengthens muscles also aids in the prevention of height loss, as well as preserving strength, flexibility and stamina. It helps you to maintain your balance and coordination, protects your bones and even safeguards your mental agility. So it's worth the effort for people of all ages.

A WELL-OILED MACHINE

When you exert yourself during exercise, your heart pumps blood through your body more efficiently, flushing out your arteries and protecting them from plaque buildup. Exercise strengthens your heart, reducing your resting pulse rate (your regular heart rate without physical exertion). Some athletes have a resting heart rate as low as 40 beats a minute, but if you get no exercise, your heart has to work harder—beating as many as 100 times a minute if you're really out of shape—to do the same thing.

SELF-PROTECTION

Research indicates that adopting a relatively active lifestyle, including exercise such as a 30-minute brisk walk every day, could prevent nearly a third of new cases of obesity and more than 40 percent of new cases of diabetes (a condition strongly linked to heart disease and strokes—see page 30). Giving your muscles a workout makes it easier for your body to process energy in the form of blood sugar, or glucose. Researchers from Scotland underlined this when they found that insulin resistance in women with a high risk of diabetes dropped by 22 percent after seven weeks on an exercise program that involved running, cycling, using a rowing machine and aerobics.

THE SECRET OF YOUTH

It is no myth that exercise helps to keep you young. Studies have shown that women who stay physically active after the age of 50 are as fit as, or even fitter than, women 20 years younger who get no exercise. And a long-term American study found that men who get in shape in middle age reduce their risk of dying over the following 20 years by almost a quarter.

Giving your muscles a workout makes it easier for your body to process energy in the form of blood sugar, or glucose.

regular exercise
can change your life

If you exercise regularly, you will experience a large number of benefits to your health. All the following advantages associated with exercise are also linked with reducing the risk of heart attacks and strokes.

- Regular exercise lowers total cholesterol levels and levels of "bad" LDL cholesterol, while boosting levels of "good" HDL cholesterol and reducing plaque buildup in your arteries.
- It keeps weight down and reduces body fat.
- It lowers blood pressure.
- It boosts your heart rate while you are in the process of exercising—providing a cardiovascular workout—but lowers it in the long term, meaning that your cardiac capacity and fitness improve.
- It improves circulation and breathing, so your heart and lungs work more efficiently and you get more oxygen to vital organs and tissues.
- It stabilizes blood sugar and improves glucose metabolism, thereby lowering the risk of diabetes.
- It relieves stress and anxiety (which, as you will read in Step 9, is important for lowering the risk of heart disease).
- It boosts mood and reduces depression by releasing endorphins, the body's natural feel-good chemicals. And it may also improve any decline in mental alertness associated with depression.
- It helps you to sleep better.

Keeping physically active offers these additional benefits:

- It halves the risk of hip fracture among people over 45 and combats the crippling bone disease osteoporosis, reducing your chance of disability and dependence in old age.
- It reduces the risk of breast, bowel and lung cancer.
- It boosts general fitness, muscular strength and endurance.
- It enhances flexibility and balance.
- It tones your body, so you look better.
- It reduces the risk of erectile dysfunction in men.
- It lowers your risk of respiratory disease.

And, above all, it may prolong your life—so there's no reason why we shouldn't all make an effort to get in shape.

stand up
and stay healthy

Sitting for long periods – as many of us with sedentary jobs or inactive lifestyles tend to do – may be a health hazard, disrupting the way our bodies should function, recent scientific studies suggest. In fact, even spending an hour at the gym doesn't cancel out the effects of sitting down for hours every day.

SITTING SYNDROME

Many of us have deskbound jobs. And we also tend to sit down while relaxing— whether we're watching television or DVDs, playing video games or chatting with friends online.

What makes sitting for long periods so hazardous, say researchers, is that, while sitting, we don't even make the normal brief but frequent muscular contractions that occur when standing or walking. These small, intermittent movements may be necessary to keep our bodies in good working order.

For instance, when we are sedentary for too long, certain chemicals in the body that play a part in burning fat stop functioning. An enzyme called lipase which, when we are engaged in activity, helps muscles to round up fats circulating in the bloodstream, virtually shuts down when we sit down. With nowhere else to go, blood fats either stick in artery linings, causing the buildup of plaque, or are stored as body fat. And sitting for long periods reduces levels

Action station Dr. James Levine of the Mayo Clinic has developed a desk that can be used without sitting down. It is built on the principle of a treadmill, to which, if you prefer, you can add an exercise ball to sit on while you work. He claims that, compared with sitting in a chair, people burn an extra 100 Cal an hour walking while they work – equivalent to a weight loss of 56 lb a year if they use the desk for eight hours daily. The adjustable model (left) is a version from TrekDesk, which fits onto an existing treadmill.

of "good" HDL cholesterol by almost one quarter, increasing the risk of heart problems and metabolic diseases such as diabetes. This may explain why light activity has been shown to reduce levels of blood sugar.

ON YOUR FEET

By contrast, every two hours we spend standing or walking around at home reduces our risk of obesity by 9 percent and diabetes by 12 percent, according to the results of a study by Dr. Frank Hu, an expert in nutrition at Harvard School of Public Health. Standing burns an extra 60 Cal an hour compared with sitting. That may not seem like much, but over an eight-hour working day that's 480 Cal—or roughly 33 pounds in a 46-week working year. So if you habitually sit instead of stand, you need to either reduce what you eat by an equivalent amount, or burn off that many more calories through activity. Dr. Hu's prescription for a healthy lifestyle is to do at least half an hour of brisk walking every day and to limit the time you spend watching television to ten hours a week. It is as important to decrease sedentary behaviour, especially watching television, as it is to do more physical activity, he says. Dr. Hu's personal solution is to have a treadmill in front of the television, so he can exercise while watching the news.

MOVE YOUR MUSCLES

If you are obliged to sit for prolonged periods, try to change position regularly. You could also exercise your legs under the desk, stretch your neck, shoulders and arms, wriggle in your chair, clench your buttocks and abdominal muscles— anything that gets parts of your body moving that would otherwise be still. Most importantly, you should get up and move around at regular intervals. Take a short break every hour, if you can, and do something active—even if it's simply walking to the photocopier, or doing sit-ups or jumping-jacks during commericals while you watch TV.

defeat **deskbound** disease

Whether you work from home or in an office, you can fight off the afflictions that come from sitting at a desk for hours at a time. Try the routines described below. You will find that they relieve tension and stress, and ease headaches and tiredness.

- **Neck tilt** Keeping your shoulders loose and your face turned forward, lean your head toward your shoulder on one side then the other. Bend your head forward to touch your chin to your chest, then gently lean it back as far as you comfortably can. Repeat sequence twice.
- **Shoulder roll** Raise your shoulders as high as they will go and roll them forward and backward until you feel the tension release.
- **Chest expansion** Clasp your hands behind your head and pull your elbows backward, moving your shoulder blades together. Repeat three times.
- **Arm stretch** Push your arms out straight to the sides, palms up, as far as they will go, then bend your arms and touch your shoulders with your fingertips. Release.
- **Arm strengthening** Sit in a chair with firm armrests. Sit normally with your feet on the floor and place your palms on the armrests, pushing yourself up with your hands as if getting up from the chair. Hold when your legs are almost straight, then slowly lower yourself. Repeat twice on the first day, four times on the second and so on, aiming for ten repetitions in total.
- **Wrist pull** Keeping your shoulders relaxed, make a fist with one hand and flex it inwards as far as you can toward your forearm. Press your fist gently with the other hand and hold for 3 seconds. End by circling your wrist and clenched fist inwards and outwards three times. Relax and do the same on the other side, then repeat the whole sequence.
- **Back stretch** Fold your arms across your chest until your hands reach as far behind your back on the opposite side as possible, as if trying to hug yourself. Hold for 10 seconds, then repeat with the opposite arm on top. Next, place your palms in the small of your back, elbows out, and arch your back forward, pulling your shoulder blades inwards. Hold for 3 seconds and relax.
- **Thigh stretch** Place one foot on top of the opposite knee, then bend forward to touch your forehead on your knee. Repeat on the other side.
- **Leg lift** Sitting with your feet away from your desk, stretch your legs out as far as you can and raise each one in turn until it lifts your thigh away from your chair. Repeat ten times on each side.

the key to **motivation**

Since everyday modern life is relatively sedentary, most of us who want to improve our fitness have to make conscious decisions to be more physically active. The strength of your motivation will make a huge difference to how successful you are.

In general, formulating positive reasons for taking exercise is far more effective than dwelling on negative ones, according to psychologists. So if you are thinking about starting to do regular exercise because someone close to you has had a heart attack, try to reframe this as a positive wish to stay healthy and have lots of energy. People who are strongly motivated tend to exercise more and to persist for longer than those who are not—and they are more likely to enjoy it. You may feel more tired and stressed out than you used to be, have aches and pains that you didn't used to have, or simply not feel as healthy as you once did. The trick is to harness these complaints into positive long-term incentives for exercising, such as wanting to get in shape, sleep better or maintain your muscle strength and stay independent as you get older.

And remember that the longer you can keep going with your exercise program, the more likely it is that healthy exercise will become a permanent part of your life.

SECRETweapon

EXERCISE BUDDY

You can increase your chances of sticking to an exercise program by making a deal with a friend to go for a walk together every week at a set time, or by joining a walking group. Studies show that people who undertake activities with a spouse, partner, friend or in a class are more motivated. If you make a firm commitment, you are much less likely to change your mind because it's raining or because you just feel too tired.

EXERCISE THAT FITS INTO YOUR LIFESTYLE

Some people believe that only intense or structured exercise, such as aerobics, counts as a cardiovascular workout—but it is the total amount of activity in your daily life that matters most. As the World Health Organization points out, there are four major "domains" in most people's days—work, travel, home and leisure—and there are opportunities for physical activity during all of them. Exercise that fits into your lifestyle can be more effective than structured exercise. So perhaps the key is to abolish the "E" word altogether, and just think about how, when and where in the course of your everyday life you can add more physical activities. Try to find opportunities for activity throughout the day, every day.

Richard Winterflood

The runner

Richard Winterflood took up running when he returned to
university. "Hours of studying books alone in a small room left
me with an overpowering desire to get out into the open air. I
was an enthusiastic athlete when I was younger and my body
seemed to need it," he says.

"The exercise itself is a source of great pleasure: the
enhanced feeling of well-being, greater mental alertness, the
awareness that you can undertake all sorts of physical activity
or respond to physical challenges," says Richard. "But also, as
I run throughout the year, it is the increased awareness of
nature - the cycle of birth, growth, fruition and death
witnessed in gardens, yards and parks."

"The exercise itself is a source of great
pleasure," says Richard, "the enhanced feeling of
well-being, greater mental alertness ..."

Now retired, Richard runs every day early in the morning.
"As I've grown fitter and leaner, I run with greater ease.
Increasingly, as my body takes over the basic rhythm of the
running, my mind is left free to scan the path ahead, the choice
of paths between the trees, the speed with which I feel I want
to run, the kind of step I want to use. The rhythmic variation
links with my mood and what I'm thinking and feeling."

What also makes him happy is that his enthusiasm appears to
be infectious. "Some months ago a wiry middle-aged man
exercising on a set of parallel bars in the forest called out
and told me that he'd watched me and was now following my
exercise example - albeit in his own way."

More recently during his daily runs, he noticed that an
older denim-clad man whom he'd seen for years regularly walking
his dog was suddenly absent. Where was he, Richard wondered?

"Six months earlier, he had told me that his dog was getting
too old to give him any real exercise," says Richard. "Recently,
I've glimpsed him twice, the first time walking - without his
dog. Then a few days later, I saw him again - running and still
in his habitual denim. I couldn't help smiling as I watched him
disappear through the trees."

MAKE IT EASY

Here are a few simple psychological incentives to increase your motivation and help you stay on track:

- **Change your mindset** Don't think, "I should exercise." Think, "a quick stroll now would clear my head," or "a swim in the morning would give me more energy for the day."
- **Do something you enjoy** Some people love going to the gym; others feel intimidated by all the equipment. Some feel motivated if they take classes with other people; others prefer jogging solo. Some people are most energetic first thing in the morning; others are better in the afternoon. Make your chosen activity fit your personality and lifestyle.
- **Start small** If you find exercise hard, start by doing just 10 minutes on three days a week—then 15 minutes, then four times a week, and so on. Take at least one day off from your routine each week.
- **Make exercise fit into your routine** If you have to travel a long way to get to where you exercise, at a time of day that makes it hard to fit in with other commitments, you'll probably give up in a week. Schedule activity at a convenient place and time.
- **Get the right clothing** Choose loose, comfortable clothes for exercising. If you decide to go running, get proper footwear; nothing undermines exercise plans faster than pain or injury. If it boosts your confidence, buy some attractive running gear or a new bathing suit.

before you start running

Jogging is a very effective way to achieve cardiovascular fitness and burn calories, but you have to start slowly, particularly if you haven't done any running before. Make sure that you follow these guidelines:

- Buy a comfortable pair of good running shoes that cushion and support your feet. You should buy a new pair every six months if you run regularly.
- Always warm up and stretch thoroughly before you start (see page 155).
- Take things slowly at first—for instance, start by walking most of the way, then gradually include periods of jogging. As you become fitter, you can gradually increase the time you run.
- You will need to breathe a little harder (to get more oxygen into your body), but you should still be able to talk to a friend while you jog. If you can't, you might be overdoing it. If you get uncomfortably winded, slow down or walk until you recover
- Bear in mind that, although jogging is less stressful than sprinting, it is still a relatively high-impact activity and not always suitable for people with knee or ankle problems.

- **Stick to the schedule** If you can't face a 30-minute workout, don't just sink into the nearest armchair—go for a walk instead. But keep to your routine. If it starts to rain right when you had planned to go for a bike ride through the park, vacuum the living room or clean the windows instead (yes, housework does count—see page 166).
- **Be honest** Don't fall back on the excuse that you are "too busy" to do exercise. Think about how much time you spend sitting during the day: Americans spend about three hours a day watching TV, and Statistics Canada puts average Canadian TV time at about 2.1 hours a day. If you're really strapped for time, spread activity into shorter bursts throughout the day.

BEFORE YOU START

Although most of us do need to get more exercise, people who have been inactive for a while may have health concerns about embarking on an exercise program. If any of the following applies to you, you should talk to your doctor before starting:

- You have had a heart attack or stroke.
- You have heart disease or diabetes, or are seriously overweight.
- You have asthma, or lung, liver or kidney disease.
- You have osteoporosis or arthritis, or have had joint surgery.
- You have had a recent joint, muscle, tendon or ligament injury.
- You have balance problems or dizzy spells.
- You are a man aged over 45 or a woman over 55 with high blood pressure or high cholesterol.

If you haven't exercised for a considerable length of time, it is important to start slowly and build it up gradually. First, think about adding some walking and gentle stretching exercises to your daily routine, or going swimming with a friend a couple of times a week. If you do join a gym, ask the trainer to help you to plan a program tailored to your own starting fitness level (your resting pulse rate—see page 144—is an indication).

TALK TO YOUR DOCTOR

Starting an exercise program can be especially difficult if you have mobility problems. If you have had a stroke or are recovering after a heart attack, discuss your plan with your doctor or rehabilitation specialist.

I have angina. Will exercise increase my risk of a heart attack?

Yes and no. In people with severe blockages of the arteries supplying the heart muscle, activities such as push-ups or weight lifting can increase the stress on the heart to the point where it might lead to a heart attack. On the other hand, regular gentle aerobic exercise—such as walking or swimming—should help your angina, making a heart attack less likely in the long term.

GENTLY ON THE JOINTS

Gentle exercise has been shown to improve symptoms of arthritis. It can reduce joint pain and stiffness, help build the muscles that support your joints, improve flexibility and increase endurance. Of course, exercise also helps control your weight, taking the load off your knee joints, and it can reduce the risk of other skeletal problems such as osteoporosis.

Compared to brisk walking, strolling reduces the strain on knee joints by around 25 percent, helping to burn calories while reducing the risk of injury. In Nordic walking (see page 169), the poles take the weight off your joints and you burn more calories per mile. Swimming or tai chi are also good options for safe, low-impact aerobic workouts.

Always begin an exercise routine slowly, increasing the intensity and pace as your muscles warm up. If you find even gentle exercises too painful at first, try a water exercise program (your local pool probably runs one). The buoyancy of your body in water reduces the stress on your hips, knees and spine, making movement easier.

HOW MUCH EXERCISE DO YOU NEED?

To gain cardiovascular benefits, you need to do at least 30 minutes of moderate-intensity exercise five days a week. (Moderate-intensity exercise makes you feel slightly warm and slightly out of breath.) If you find this daunting, then begin with 10 minutes three times a day and gradually build up to an unbroken 30 minutes.

simple **workout** routines

There are two types of exercise: aerobic and isometric. Aerobic exercise gets your heart beating faster and your lungs working harder. Isometric exercise—also known as resistance training or weight training—builds muscles by making them lift, pull or move something heavy. The classic way to weight train is with weights at a gym, but you can also do simple exercises using portable dumbbells. An ideal exercise plan incorporating both types of exercise consists of the following components:

- A warm-up at the start of each session to help to loosen your muscles, tendons and ligaments, and to prevent injury.
- Stretching exercises to increase flexibility, improve the range of motion of your joints, enhance posture and boost circulation.
- Aerobic exercise to improve stamina and build cardiovascular strength. Examples include brisk walking, running, swimming, biking, dancing and certain household or gardening chores. To be effective, the activity should last for about 20 minutes.
- Weight training through resistance exercises, to maintain and enhance muscle mass and strength, and help burn calories more efficiently.
- Exercises for core muscles in your lower back, abdomen and pelvis, to enhance balance and stability.

EXERCISE AIDS

Two pieces of inexpensive equipment can help you to build strong muscles and a healthy heart: an exercise ball and dumbbells. You can buy them at department stores, supermarkets and sports equipment stores.

A large inflated stability ball is particularly good for strength-training exercises. You have to work hard to stay balanced when sitting on the ball, so you use all your muscles, especially those in your core—your abdomen, back and hips. Exercise balls are beneficial to good posture and coordination too. Make sure you buy the right size for your height. Most balls have size charts. For example, people who are between 5 ft, 3 in and 6 ft tall should buy a 25 in (65 cm) ball.

When using a ball for the first time, practice getting comfortable by putting your back against a wall and placing your feet wide apart to make balancing easier. Then move the ball away from the wall and progress to putting your hand out for support. As you start to feel more stable, take your hand away and practice sitting with your arms raised to the sides, then overhead. To work more exercise into your day, try sitting on a balance ball while watching television. (You can buy a base for the ball to keep it stationary if this type of exercise is new to you.)

Dumbbells help to build muscle. Use a lighter pair for arm strengthening exercises and a heavier pair for leg strengthening exercises. Women should aim to use weights in the 4–22 lb (1.5–10 kg) range; men, in the 11–33 lb (5–15 kg) range.

basic stretching exercises

Stretching before exercise helps to prevent injury and keeps you flexible, making it easier to do many physical activities. Here are four simple stretches: a calf stretch, hamstring stretch, lower-back stretch and quadriceps stretch.

CALF STRETCH

Take a step forward with your right foot. Keeping your left leg straight and both heels on the ground, lean forward. You will feel a stretch in your Achilles tendon, at the back of your foot, and your calf muscles. Repeat with the other leg.

HAMSTRING STRETCH

Place your left heel on a low stool, step or anything you have on hand, such as an upturned bucket. Put your hands above your hips for support. Bend over very slowly, keeping your back straight and shoulders square until you feel a stretch at the back of your leg. Repeat with the other leg.

LOWER-BACK STRETCH

Lie on your back with your knees bent. Using both hands, pull your left knee to your chest, pressing your lower back into the floor. You should feel the stretch in your buttocks and lower back. Repeat with the right knee.

QUADRICEPS STRETCH

Place your right hand on a chair or against a wall for balance. Hold your left foot with your left hand and pull your foot gently toward your buttocks, keeping your standing leg slightly bent. You should feel a stretch in the muscle at the front of your thigh. Repeat with the right foot.

Aerobic exercise is an excellent way to burn body fat.

NO PAIN, NO GAIN

It is not true that exercise needs to hurt to be effective. If you are doing enough to benefit your health and burn up calories, you will feel warmer than usual, your breathing will be quicker and your heart rate slightly raised. If you're not generally very active, your muscles may feel a little sore and stiff the day after exercise, but actual muscle pain during exercise means that you are overdoing it and you need to slow down. So you don't want to "feel the burn," no matter what anybody says. If you develop any of these symptoms during exercise, stop what you're doing and call your doctor right away:

- Pain in your chest, arms or jaw.
- Shortness of breath that lasts for more than 10 minutes, even after you stop exercising.
- Feeling faint or giddy.
- Heart palpitations.
- Breaking out in a cold sweat.
- Nausea or vomiting.

AEROBIC EXERCISE

During aerobic exercise, your breathing gets deeper as you bring more oxygen into your lungs. Your pulse speeds up as your heart pumps blood faster around your body. Your blood vessels dilate to allow more oxygenated blood into your muscles. This is an excellent way to burn fat and lose weight, reducing stress on bones and muscles.

Your heart and the muscles around your lungs respond to aerobic exercise by getting stronger. Your body uses the oxygen it takes in during exercise to convert the energy stored as sugars and fats into usable physical energy. In this way, the more exercise you do, the more fat you burn off.

Any exercise that raises your heart rate will benefit your cardiovascular system and help you lose weight, as long as it is performed frequently and at the

exercise and heart rate

We all have a maximum heart rate, above which we are overexerting our hearts and putting ourselves at risk. For most people, the maximum heart rate is 220 minus your age. So, if you are 50, your maximum heart rate is 170 beats per minute.

Doctors and fitness experts recommend that, during exercise, people should reach and maintain roughly 60 to 65 percent of their maximum heart rates—and, to promote good health, this level of exertion should be maintained for at least 30 minutes a day. For a 50 year old, this would be 102 beats per minute. In comparison, the average person has a resting heart rate of about 70 beats per minute.

You can measure your heart rate yourself, either manually or by using a special monitor. If you want to do it manually, start by checking your resting heart rate by counting your pulse for a minute (see page 67). Then do the same again after exercise, to see how close you are to reaching your maximum.

correct intensity. Popular activities include running, cycling, rowing, playing soccer, racket sports like tennis, organized aerobics classes and gym-based workouts using equipment such as steppers.

If you are devising your own aerobic-exercise program, structure each session as follows: about 10 minutes warming up, 10 to 20 minutes exercising and 5 to 10 minutes cooling down. Build up to exercising three to five times a week. (See page 158 for a range of aerobic exercises.)

ISOMETRIC EXERCISE

Isometric exercise produces muscle tension without moving the joint and increases strength, but does not benefit the cardiovascular system immediately. It is not suitable for some people with heart disease or high blood pressure.

But this form of exercise can prevent the loss of muscle mass that often accompanies aging and may stop the decline in metabolism that leads to "middle-age spread." Simply having more muscle on your body means that you burn more calories. In women, it can also increase bone density and help prevent osteoporosis.

REDalert

WEIGHT LIMITS

In contrast to aerobics, which exercises your heart and cardiovascular system, isometric exercise, or weight training, is a form of activity designed to exercise your muscles. Using weights is a good way to maintain and build muscle mass, but it's important not to try to lift weights that are too heavy, since this can put stress on your heart and increase blood pressure. So this is one instance where you can't necessarily incorporate exercise into everyday tasks by, for example, lifting big sacks of potatoes. People who already have heart disease or high blood pressure should not do heavy isometric exercises.

an aerobics program
ten exercises

If you want to try an aerobics program at home, try the exercises described here. You may not be able to do all of them every day, but you should do them when you can. Some, such as the star jump, are fairly demanding, but there are also simple bends and strides that you should be able to work into your daily routine.

1 Spot jog Lift your knees to waist height as you jog on the spot. Keep your stomach tight and land on your toes. Jog continuously for 30 seconds.

2 Star thrust Squat on your toes with your hands on the floor just over shoulder-width apart. Keep your stomach tight and your back straight. Jump your feet back so that your legs are extended behind you in a push-up position. Jump your feet forward into the squat position again, and move back up into standing position. Repeat continuously for 30 seconds.

3 Bridge Lie on your back with your legs bent and your feet flat on the floor. Place your hands flat on the ground beside your body. Exhale as you use your abdominal muscles to push your buttocks up and away from the mat, straightening your body. Inhale as you come back down. Repeat continuously for 30 seconds.

4 Speedball Bend your arms at 90 degrees and hold them in front of you at chest level. Circle your arms around each other continuously for 15 seconds. Change direction and circle them for another 15 seconds.

5 Star jump Bend into a squat, then jump straight up. As you jump, open your legs wide and move your arms up and out, so that your body forms a star shape. Move down into a squat position as you land, ready to jump again. Repeat continuously for 30 seconds.

6 Side stride Stand with your feet together, your hands on your hips and your back straight. Step sideways with your right foot, then follow with your left foot so your feet are together. Step back to the side with your left foot and follow with your right foot. Repeat continuously for 30 seconds.

7 Lunge Stand with your feet together. Inhale and take a large step forward. As your foot touches the floor, bend your knee and lower your body until your leg is at a 90-degree angle. Exhale and push yourself back up to standing. Alternate legs continuously for 30 seconds.

8 Side jump Stand with your feet together. Imagine a straight line on the ground heading away from you. With your feet together and your knees slightly bent, jump from one side of the line to the other. Repeat continuously for 30 seconds.

9 Wall push-up Stand facing a wall, about an arm's length away from it. Place your palms flat on the wall at shoulder height and slightly wider than shoulder-width apart. Inhale as you bend your arms, leaning your body in toward the wall. Keep your stomach tight and your back straight. Exhale as you push yourself back up to the starting position. Repeat continuously for 30 seconds.

10 Cross jump Stand with your feet together. Imagine that you are standing in the center of a cross with one line extending in front and behind you, and the other out to your sides. With your feet together and knees slightly bent, jump forward along the imaginary line, then back to the center point. Jump backward along the line, then return to the center. Jump out to the right and return, and out to the left and return. Repeat continuously for 30 seconds.

weight training

By building muscle mass, weight training is the best long-term strategy for burning more calories and reducing body fat. The isometric exercises below require a few inexpensive items: dumbbells, a stability ball and an exercise mat (see "Exercise aids," page 154).

BACK AND BICEPS

1 Back fly Sit on the edge of a stability ball or chair with your feet flat on the floor. Hold a dumbbell in each hand. Keeping your back flat, bend forward at the waist and lower your chest to about 3–4 in (7–10 cm) above your knees, letting your arms hang down on either side of your legs with your hands by your feet. Squeeze your shoulder blades and raise the weights out to the side until your arms are outstretched parallel with the floor. Pause, then slowly return to the starting position.

2 Bent-over row Stand with your feet shoulder-width apart, your back straight and your knees slightly bent for support. Hold a dumbbell in each hand. Keeping your back straight, bend 90 degrees from the waist and let your arms hang toward the floor, palms facing your legs. Squeeze your shoulder blades together and bend your elbows, raising the dumbbells on either side of your body, as if rowing. Pause, then slowly return to the starting position.

CHEST AND TRICEPS

1 Stability-ball push-up Place a stability ball against a wall, then kneel in front of it so that it is between you and the wall. Place your hands on the ball so they are directly below your shoulders. Walk back on your knees until your body forms a straight line from your head to your knees. You should be leaning forward into the ball. Keeping your torso straight and your abdominal muscles contracted (concentrate on pulling your belly button toward your spine), bend your elbows and lower your chest toward the ball. Stop when your elbows are in line with your shoulders. Pause, then return to the starting position.

160

2 Triceps pushback Sit on a stability ball with your knees bent and your feet flat on the floor. Hold the dumbbells in front of you with your arms bent at a 90-degree angle and your elbows at your sides. Keeping your back straight, bend slightly from the hips. Straighten your arms and extend the weights behind your back, turning your palms toward the ceiling once your arms are fully extended. Pause, then return to the starting position.

LEGS AND CORE

1 Side plank Lie on your left side with your knees bent. Bend your left arm so your forearm is extended in front of you perpendicular to your body, then lift your torso off the floor. Your upper body should form a straight line from your hips to your shoulders. Place your right hand on your hip and hold for 5 to 15 seconds. Return to the starting position, then repeat on other side. Work up to holding on each side for 30 to 60 seconds.

2 Hover Lie facing the floor with your upper body propped on your forearms. Your elbows should be directly beneath your shoulders and your palms flat on the floor. Raise your body so that your torso, hips and legs are off the floor and your body is in a straight line, supported on your forearms and toes. Don't let your back arch or droop, and hold for 10 to 20 seconds.

Walk up and down stairs whenever you can.

find time for fitness

It is often difficult to find time to fit exercise into a busy schedule. There is a tendency to think that, if you can't do the recommended daily minimum of 30 minutes, there is no point in doing any exercise at all. In many surveys, lack of time is the main excuse people give for not being more active. But bear in mind that you don't have to do it all at once. You can achieve your daily quota by breaking it up into three shorter bursts of exercise lasting 10 minutes each. The trick is to build activity into your everyday life.

BOOSTING DAILY ACTIVITY

Here are some ways in which you can boost your daily level of activity when you just don't have time for a traditional exercise regime:

- Get up half an hour earlier once a week. Use the extra time to do some floor exercises (getting an exercise DVD can help), or go for a walk or swim. Once you're happy with that, do it twice a week.
- Walk up and down stairs whenever you can. If you use an elevator at work, get out two floors below your usual level. Walking up just two flights of stairs a day can add up to 6 lb of weight loss over a year.
- During lunch break at work, instead of eating at your desk or sitting in the staff cafeteria, have a quick snack and go for a walk outside.
- Get off the bus one stop earlier than usual and walk the rest of the way.
- Park a little further away than you really need to each time you arrive at the office or go shopping, and walk the rest of the way. From time to time, increase the distance and try to walk a little faster.
- Think about how to incorporate activity into your regular routine. Could you bike to the store, for example, or swap your regular trip to the movie theater for a bowling or ice-skating session?
- Treat waiting times as opportunities for action. Don't simply stare at your computer screen while waiting for a page to load; do a quick arm stretch

or three. Waiting for the kettle to boil? Try a few squats, holding the edge of the countertop or the back of a kitchen chair, if necessary.

- While watching television, make sure you spend at least 10 minutes out of each hour doing something else as well, such as sit-ups or stretching exercises. Getting up during the commercials to load the dishwasher and tidy the kitchen can add up to 15 minutes of activity every hour.
- Do the ironing while watching a movie, or set up an exercise bike or treadmill in front of the television. In 10 minutes, you'll burn 62 Cal ironing or 97 Cal on the bike or treadmill.

take the high-intensity route

Busy workers with little time for exercise may be heartened by a recent small Scottish study that concluded that short bursts of intense exercise every few days could dramatically reduce the risk of certain diseases.

"Many people feel they simply don't have the time to follow current guidelines on exercise," says Dr. James Timmons, one of the study's researchers. These guidelines recommend that we perform moderate to vigorous aerobic and resistance (isometric) exercise several hours a week. "The risk of cardiovascular disease or Type 2 diabetes is greatly reduced by regular physical activity," says Timmons, "but we also found that short bursts of exercise can be highly beneficial."

The researchers studied 25 inactive men, each of whom did four to six 30-second sessions on an exercise bike, going as fast as they could and taking 4 minutes of rest between each sprint. They did this three times a week for two weeks. The result—based on a total of just 15 minutes of intensive exercise over the course of a fortnight—was a 23 percent improvement in insulin sensitivity, demonstrated by the speed at which the subjects' bodies removed glucose from the bloodstream after exercise.

The explanation for this is that intense muscle contraction is the only way to remove glycogen—the body's stored form of glucose—from muscles.

"Think about diabetes as being glucose circulating in the blood rather than stored in the muscles where it should be," says Dr. Timmons. "If we take out the glycogen from the muscles through exercise, then the muscles draw in that excess glucose from the blood." He recommends four all-out 30-second sprints on an exercise bike three times a week. You could get similar benefits, he says, by running up and down four flights of stairs three times, twice a week. This exercise routine, known as "high-intensity interval training," or HIT, can work for men and women of all ages.

exercise **to suit yourself**

The favorite way for most people to get exercise is through brisk walking. In a recent survey of popular physical activities, walking came in at the top, followed by swimming, going to the gym and cycling. Jogging ranked just above golf, while aerobics was low on the list.

Walking for half an hour just three times a week is one of the best forms of exercise, offering significant benefits to cardiovascular health. Researchers studied 106 adults aged 40 to 61 who were healthy but inactive. Two groups were asked to do 30 minutes of brisk walking on either three or five days per week, while a third group did not change their activity level.

After 12 weeks, the walkers in both active groups recorded significant drops in their blood pressure and waist and hip circumference, as well as improvements in their overall level of fitness. There were no changes among the control group.

WALK TALL

If you are not used to doing much walking, start slowly and gradually pick up your pace after the first minute or two. Keep your shoulders back and relaxed and your abdomen tucked in to protect your lower back. The best rhythm and stride are the ones that feel most comfortable. If you want to increase your pace, take short quick strides—your feet will more easily get into a rhythm and you will move at a faster speed.

HOW MANY STEPS DO YOU TAKE?

A pedometer is a cheap step-counting device that is very useful if you are trying to increase your overall level of daily activity. Just strap one on to your waistband and go about your life. It's a simple way of measuring just how active you are. You won't be able to resist taking a look at your step count—and that could inspire you to increase it.

If you are fairly inactive, you probably take around 3,000 steps a day. An average daily level is 7,000 steps for men and 5,000 steps for women. In trials, people wearing pedometers take an average of 2,491 more steps a day than people not wearing them (2,000 steps is about a mile, so that represents nearly 9 miles a week). Wearing a pedometer will increase your level of physical activity, and users also experience significant reductions in blood pressure and BMI (see page 66). Having a target number of steps to aim for has been proven to increase step counts more effectively than aiming for a 30-minute brisk walk daily. Experts recommend aiming for at least 10,000 steps a day, which will burn around 500 Cal, or 3,500 Cal over

The ideal is to complete at least 10,000 steps a day.

the course of a week. As long as you don't increase your calorie consumption, you'll lose a pound for the price of a little extra footwork. If your starting level is a lot lower than the average, simply set interim goals—5,000 steps a day, then 6,000, and so on.

The more you can do, the better. A 2008 study involving 14 researchers from around the world showed that, for effective weight control, women under 40 and men under 50 should aim for as many as 12,000 steps a day.

WANT TO JOIN A GYM?

If you want to become a member of a gym or health center but feel too embarrassed to make the first move, take a friend with you. Most gyms will

Building up your muscle power could increase your life span.

be strong, live long

Building up muscle power can increase a man's life span. That's the conclusion of a study in Sweden in which researchers tested the strength and fitness levels of 8,762 men aged between 20 and 80 and followed them for almost 20 years. They found that men with greater muscular strength at the outset had lower rates of death from all causes, including cancer. The strongest group of men was 23 percent less likely to have died at the end of the follow-up period than the weakest group—and it had 29 percent fewer deaths from cardiovascular disease.

be only too happy to give you a personal tour and, once you've seen the equipment and met the staff, it will seem less intimidating. It may also be a good idea to go in January, when many gyms offer special reduced rates to mark the start of a new year.

Just avoid gyms with gleaming wall-to-wall mirrors. According to researchers at McMaster University in Hamilton, Canada, exercising in front of a mirror makes women feel less energized and relaxed than exercising without a mirror. Even women who feel good about their bodies experience negative feelings after working out in front of their reflections.

home is where the heart gets healthy

Doing household chores, cleaning windows, gardening and DIY projects are among the ideal ways to increase your heart rate. They all involve NEAT, Non-Exercise Activity Thermogenesis (the heat or energy we use up in routine daily activities—see pages 137–38). Dr. James Levine of the Mayo Clinic, whose team led the reseach on NEAT, estimates that the many

Put on some lively, invigorating music.

conveniences we use daily—everything from cars and elevators, to dishwashers and television remote controls—deprive us of 100 to 200 Cal per day of NEAT that we could be expending. According to Dr. Levine, this may be the cause of "the entire obesity epidemic."

The next time you do housework, try the routine described below. It is guaranteed to get you moving up a gear.

● Put on some lively, invigorating music to keep the pace going, and sing along with it so you exercise your lungs and chest muscles.

● Start with a light chore, such as dusting, as a warm-up.

● Make a conscious effort to contract abdominal and thigh muscles when you bend and stretch (such as when making beds), holding for 10 seconds each time.

● Run up and down the stairs as often as you can. This is a wonderful aerobic workout, especially if you are carrying a heavy load.

● When you are cleaning windows or polishing, deliberately trace wide energetic loops to help tone and strengthen arm muscles.

● Push the vacuum cleaner as far forward as you can on each sweep.

● When you are picking things up to tidy a room or fill a laundry basket, do a separate squat for each item, bending from the knees and keeping your back straight.

● Use a low stool to do step-up exercises when cleaning windows or dusting shelves and picture frames.

HOUSEHOLD MUSCLE

Did you know that climbing a flight of stairs in a typical house burns 2 Cal in under 15 seconds? The table on the next page shows how you can use a little muscle and get fit, while also saving money you would have spent getting someone else to do these tasks for you. The figures represent extra calories burned, in addition to what you expend by simply existing. They are averages. The heavier you are, the more calories you burn.

Energetic gardening—a great way
to add activity to your life

household muscle

activity	Cal/hour	Cal/10 minutes
decorating/DIY projects	383	63.8
energetic gardening	340	56.7
mowing the lawn	333	55.5
mopping the floor	268	44.7
washing the car	250	41.7
weeding	248	41.3
cleaning windows	180	30
dusting	174	29
washing the dishes	171	28.5
ironing	142	23.7
standing	91	15.2

ENJOY YOURSELF

The key to staying active is doing things that are fun. Exercise doesn't have to be confined to working out in a gym or pounding the pavement, and there is a huge variety of ways to add activity to your life without seeing it as punishment. Are there any activities that you've always wanted to do but never got around to trying—such as playing golf, scuba diving or scaling a climbing wall? Here are some more ideas to inspire you:

● **Join a walking club** Walking with others is an excellent way to get fit. Being part of a club means that there are other people to socialize with and to motivate you, and you are regularly required to be present at a specific time and place. Before joining a club, find out how far the members generally walk and whether it is suitable for your current fitness level. You don't want to find yourself on a 20-mile (32-km) hike when you'd been anticipating a half-hour stroll in the park.

- **Nordic walking** Try a Scandinavian form of walking that's gaining popularity. It uses special poles to help to propel you forward, taking some of the weight off your knees and providing a great cardiovascular workout. A little like cross-country skiing, Nordic walking exercises both your upper and lower body. It uses more muscles and burns more calories than ordinary walking (while seeming to require a lot less effort), aids flexibility and helps people with balance problems.
- **Be a kid again** Children are the world's best exercise aid. They won't stay indoors because it's raining, sit down because they feel like a nap or get distracted because they're worried about a deadline. And children need exercise too, as a break from watching television and playing computer games. They make activity fun and spread their infectious enthusiasm for life. So go for a bike ride with your kids, play soccer in the park, kick leaves and splash in puddles, throw a football, fly a kite, skip, play hide-and-seek, take them to the beach … the possibilities are endless.

If there are no kids at home, how about getting a dog?

- **Get a dog** If there are no kids in your home, have you thought about getting a dog? Dogs won't put up with excuses when you don't feel like taking them for a walk, and they offer companionship and a chance to meet other dog owners. Studies show that dog owners are less stressed, get more exercise and have lower blood pressure and lower cholesterol levels than the general population. What's more, they tend to be healthier overall, with fewer minor health issues and other medical complaints.
- **Skip yourself fit** Skipping is good for the heart, bones, flexibility and coordination. Ten minutes of skipping will burn between 70 Cal and 110 Cal.
- **Get wet** If the thought of swimming endless laps without a break keeps you away from the pool, try alternating lap-swimming with a few gentle water exercises.

- **Yoga** You've heard of it, but have you tried it? Yoga can boost cardiovascular fitness, lung capacity, muscular strength and flexibility, and it's a very effective stress-reliever. One review of 70 studies worldwide showed that doing yoga regularly can reduce numerous risk factors associated with cardiovascular disease.

- **Sing your heart out** Singing exercises your heart and lungs, boosts your circulation, improves cardiovascular efficiency, increases oxygen uptake, enhances alertness and is a great workout for upper body muscles—as well as making you feel energized and more positive about yourself. Singing can also reduce pain and help people to recover from strokes and heart attacks. Even if you do it only once a month, singing can make an extraordinary difference.

- **Tai chi** This ancient Chinese technique has been described as an art form as well as a type of exercise. It involves a series of flowing, coordinated body movements sometimes known as "moving meditation," and aims to harmonize mind and body while developing flexibility, strength, balance, posture and calm. Since the movements are so gentle, tai chi is suitable for almost anyone, even people recovering from injuries or frail older people. It has been shown to be as effective as an aerobic workout in lowering blood pressure.

Singing exercises your heart and lungs, boosts your circulation and improves cardiovascular efficiency.

FIND OUT HOW IN SHAPE YOU ARE – THEN AIM HIGHER

No matter how fit you are right now and however you decide to exercise, it is good to have a goal and a way to measure your success. So, before you start, do a few checks and write down the results. Check again every six weeks, and watch as your fitness level climbs. Make your goals realistic—and be sure to reward yourself when you hit your target.

- Find out your fitness level by establishing your resting pulse rate (see page 67). Generally, the lower the rate, the fitter you are—well-trained athletes' heart rates may drop as low as 40 to 60 beats per minute. A high resting heart rate is a predictor of heart attacks and coronary death in both men and women. Aim to bring yours down.
- Take what you would consider a reasonable walk at a reasonably brisk pace. Record your pulse rate immediately afterwards and 2 minutes later; write down how far you walked and how long it took you. Your aim is to walk further and faster each week and to see your pulse return to its resting level more quickly.
- Next, look back at the various measurements you took earlier: BMI, waist and hip circumference and waist-to-hip ratio (see pages 66-67). If you are overweight, you should aim to reduce all these figures.
- If you have a pedometer, record how many steps you take during an average day of the week and on the weekend. Try to increase this number—the more steps, the better. Settle on a realistic short-term target at the start, depending on your initial step count, and aim for at least 10,000 as your final goal.
- Improve your "recovery rate." Your resting pulse rate gives you some measure of your fitness level, but for an accurate assessment you need to know how quickly your heart rate returns to normal after exercise. If you have been unable to do strenuous exercise, or if you are not in shape and are just beginning to be physically active, use the measurements you took from the self-paced walking test described above. Otherwise, do some form of short-burst exercise that noticeably increases your pulse rate, such as push-ups, skipping or star jumps for as long as you can manage, between 2 and 5 minutes (but stop if you develop any pain or discomfort). Take your pulse immediately after stopping the exercise, and again 2 minutes later.

feel good

If you manage to make physical activity part of your routine, the idea of "30 minutes a day" will no longer seem daunting. You'll start to notice improvements in your health. You will look better, feel more alert, and your energy levels will soar. You'll sleep better, too, and have an easier time managing stress. It feels good to be active, independent and healthy. Start gently, build up gradually and do it regularly, and you will reap the rewards of exercise.

self-defense plan

STEP 8

EATING WELL AND STAYING FIT ARE EXCELLENT WAYS TO PROTECT AGAINST THE WEIGHT GAIN AND INACTIVITY THAT CAN RESULT IN A HEART ATTACK OR STROKE. BUT YOU SHOULD ALSO BE AWARE OF OTHER EVERYDAY ENEMIES THAT CAN CAUSE CARDIOVASCULAR PROBLEMS. THIS STEP DEALS WITH TEN COMMON HAZARDS AND HOW TO COMBAT THEM.

Safeguard
your body

We all know how good it feels to be out in the country, away from noise and traffic, and breathing clean, fresh air. Pollution from vehicles, smoke and fumes are not only unpleasant; research suggests they could threaten cardiovascular health. Similarly, the constant rumble of heavy traffic on major roads and other loud noises can pose a threat to your heart, as can cold weather and even lack of sunshine.

Every day, our bodies are exposed to a variety of toxins in the environment, some of which are easier to escape than others. You undoubtedly know about a few of the culprits already—smoking, for example, which is especially damaging to the heart and arteries and shortens lives. Most people are much less aware of other potentially dangerous toxins, such as chemicals in the plastic packaging widely used for food and drinks.

Various types of infection can also put your arteries at risk, contributing to the body-wide inflammation that underlies the development of arterial plaque (see page 18). Colds and flu can have more serious consequences than simply keeping you in bed feeling miserable for a few days. And, while moderate consumption of alcohol, especially red wine, seems to protect against the development of cardiovascular disease, heavy drinking—especially binge drinking—can greatly increase your risk.

POISON PURGE

Step 8 explains how we can protect our arteries from ten noxious enemies that potentially threaten all of us in our daily lives, and gives an abundance of helpful advice about how to combat their harmful effects. You may not be able to change, for example, the weather, the air you breathe when you step outside or the volume of traffic noise—but there are many things you can do to limit your exposure to them.

alcohol units

In North America, guidelines define moderate drinking as no more than one serving per day if you're a woman (or up to seven per week), and no more than two per day for a man (up to 14 per week). In Canada, the standard drink includes 13.6 g of pure alcohol, while an American standard drink includes 14 g.

A standard drink is:

 5 oz (142 mL) of wine
 12 oz (340 mL) of regular-strength beer
 1.5 oz (42.6 mL) of hard liquor

no.1 excess alcohol

Drinking a glass or two of red wine every few days can provide you with some protection against cardiovascular disease—but don't overdo it, since drinking too much will increase your risk of a heart attack or stroke.

Drinking has been on a slight upward trend in North America over the past decade and a half, according to both Statistics Canada and the US National Institute on Alcohol Abuse and Alcoholism (NIAAA). It's easy to underestimate how much you're drinking because bars and restaurants often serve drinks that exceed the standard sizes. For example, the table above shows the standard servings across both countries, but a pint of beer (16 fl oz/473 mL in the United States; 20 imperial oz/568 mL in Canada) easily surpasses the standard drink size. And of course, most bars and restaurants offer doubles of hard liquor. Remember that the next time you order drinks.

BEWARE OF BINGE DRINKING

Consuming little or no alcohol during the week does *not* mean you can "save up" for Friday night. Binge drinking—irregular bouts of heavy consumption—is especially dangerous for your heart and increases your risk of a stroke. Each episode causes a surge in blood pressure. If you do it regularly, you may develop high blood pressure which is especially likely to promote atherosclerosis, doubling your risk of a heart attack. If you regularly consume six or more servings at a single sitting (that is, within a six-hour period), you are twice as likely to have a stroke as a non-drinker.

According to the NIAAA, binge drinking is when men have five or more drinks, or women drink four or more, in two hours. In Canada, consuming at least five alcoholic drinks at one sitting is considered bingeing.

About 75 percent of the alcohol consumed in the US is imbibed during binge drinking, with half of all binge drinkers aged 18 to 20. In Canada, 24 percent of men and 7 percent of women binge drink at least once a month. If you regularly drink enough to be intoxicated, you increase your risk of dangerously abnormal heart rhythms, heart failure, strokes and sudden death—even if you have no preexisting heart disease.

TIPS FOR STAYING SOBER

Have something to eat before you go out—food slows the process of alcohol entering the bloodstream. Pace yourself: Drink slowly and alternate alcohol with water. Order light or low-alcohol beers. If you drink hard liquor, take single shots with plenty of mixer. Need an excuse? Say you're driving or taking meds.

REDalert

ALCOHOL AND YOU

If you're wondering if your drinking has crossed the line, answer the following questions:

- Have you ever felt you should cut down on your drinking?
- Have people annoyed you by criticizing your drinking?
- Have you ever felt bad or guilty about your drinking?
- Have you ever had a drink first thing in the morning to steady your nerves or get rid of a hangover?

One "yes" answer suggests a possible alcohol problem. More than one "yes" answer means it is highly likely that a problem exists. If you think that you or someone you know might have an alcohol problem, it is important to see a doctor or other health care provider right away. They can help you determine if a drinking problem exists and plan the best course of action.

no.2 gum disease

Gum disease—a chronic inflammation of the gums known medically as periodontal disease—has been shown to have a strong association with atherosclerosis. For example, a study in which samples of dental plaque (the sticky substance that accumulates on teeth) were taken from 659 people with an average age of 69 revealed that those with higher levels of four bacteria known to cause periodontal disease had thicker arterial walls in the carotid arteries supplying the brain. This sign of atherosclerosis is a strong predictor of the risk of strokes and heart attacks.

DENTAL HYGIENE

Good dental hygiene combined with regular dental checkups is the key to controlling gum disease. Brush with fluoride toothpaste for at least 2 minutes twice a day, floss daily (or use a small interdental brush) and visit your dentist every six months. It would also be a good idea to invest in an antibacterial mouthwash that reduces plaque, and a dental hygienist can remove "calcified" or hardened plaque around your teeth and below your gums.

If you are not sure whether you are cleaning your teeth effectively, ask your dentist or hygienist to check or buy chewable disclosing tablets, which leave a temporary stain on any areas of plaque and indicate where you need to clean more thoroughly. The aim is to make sure that dental plaque doesn't build up on your teeth, which also reduces the risk of sclerotic plaque building up in your arteries.

In one study, researchers in Australia and Norway tested the blood of their subjects for blood-clot risk factors and inflammation before and after dental treatment. They noted a marked reduction in risk factors after treatment, which strongly suggests that eliminating advanced gum disease could effectively reduce the risk of heart attacks or strokes. People with severe periodontal disease are almost four times as likely to have had a heart attack as those with no evidence of the disease. And recent research indicates that having extensive gum disease also doubles your risk of diabetes.

EARLY WARNINGS

Older people, smokers, tooth-grinders and those under stress have an increased risk of gum disease. Early treatment can guard against future damage to arteries, so learn to spot the warning signs.

FLOSSING MADE EASIER

When flossing your teeth, keep to a regular pattern. Start at the top and work from left to right, then move to the bottom. At first it helps to look in the mirror. Here is a good set of guidelines for flossing:

- Break off a length of floss that's about equal to the distance from your hand to your shoulder, or about 18 in (46 cm).

- Wrap most of the floss around one of your middle fingers. Then wrap the remainder around the other middle finger, leaving about 2 in (5 cm) of floss between the two. Hold the floss firmly between your thumbs and index fingers.

- Slide the floss between your teeth. When it reaches the gum line, wrap it into a C shape around the base of the tooth, just under the gumline. Then gently rub the tooth in an up--and-down motion two or three times.

- Repeat for the other side of the tooth, then the rest of the teeth, including the back sides of the last molars. As you go, wind the floss onto the finger with less floss as it picks up particles and begins to fray.

These include:

- Red, swollen or bleeding gums.
- Gums that bleed when you clean your teeth or floss.
- Loose teeth and/or gaps appearing between teeth.
- Gums receding, so teeth look longer.
- Bad breath.
- A metallic taste in your mouth.
- A change in the bite of your teeth or in the fit of partial dentures.

YOUR DENTIST

It is important to keep appointments for checkups as often as your dentist recommends to make sure any subtle changes that can herald periodontal diseases, such as inflammation of the gums (gingivitis), are picked up quickly. You should also have regular sessions with a dental hygienist, who will clean areas that it's impossible to reach by brushing and flossing alone.

no.3 smoking

Both the American Heart Association and the Heart and Stroke
Foundation of Canada say quitting smoking is an important step toward
better health. In fact, quitting is probably the most important action you
can take to reduce your risk of a heart
attack. Research suggests it will also
halve your risk of stroke and add years
to your life. In the US, one in five deaths
from cardiovascular disease is linked to
smoking. And, while tobacco use causes
the early deaths of 47,000 Canadians a
year, secondhand smoke is also a risk
factor, especially for strokes.

Like most people you want to live a
long, fulfilling and active life. So if
you smoke cigarettes, consider for a
moment the extensive harm that smoking is doing to your body:

- It damages the lining of your arteries and increases the buildup of
  sticky plaque which, over time, can clog arteries throughout your body.
- It raises levels of fibrinogen and platelets in the blood, increasing the
  tendency of blood to clot.
- It causes nine in ten cases of lung cancer and increases the risk of more
  than a dozen other cancers, including cancer of the mouth, larynx,
  esophagus, liver, pancreas, stomach, kidney, bladder and cervix.
- It raises the risk of dangerous swellings of arteries, or aneurysms.
- If you also have diabetes, it heightens the risk of cardiovascular
  disease—and you are already susceptible.
- It increases the risk of developing diabetic kidney disease or peripheral
  arterial disease so severe, that they could require amputation.

troubleshooting Q&A

I don't inhale. Am I still at risk?

Unfortunately, not inhaling makes little difference. Nicotine can be absorbed through the
membranes that line the mouth as well as those in the lungs.

Can't I just cut down or switch to a lower-tar brand?

The short answer is no. Any reduction is better than none, but as long as you continue to smoke you remain at risk. Even smoking just one to five cigarettes a day increases your risk of a heart attack by 38 percent, according to the Interheart study. Smoke more, and your risk rises in direct proportion to the number of cigarettes you smoke. If you are a two-pack-a-day smoker, your risk is increased by a staggering 920 percent.

Low-tar brands contain similar levels of tar and nicotine to normal brands; the main difference between the two types lies in the filter. But research shows that people who smoke low-tar cigarettes smoke harder and more frequently to satisfy their nicotine craving. According to one study, low-tar smokers ended up inhaling about 80 percent more smoke than those who smoked normal brands and had similar levels of cancer-causing chemicals in their blood.

● It increases levels of total and "bad" LDL cholesterol, but lowers "good" HDL cholesterol.

● It promotes an outpouring of the "fight-or-flight" stress hormone adrenaline, increasing your heart rate and blood pressure, so that your heart has to work much harder.

● It exposes you to a high intake of carbon monoxide, a poisonous gas that reduces the ability of red blood cells to carry oxygen. This makes angina (chest pain during exercise) more likely.

● It changes your body shape: Smoking alters body fat distribution to a less healthy pattern with more abdominal fat and a higher waist-to-hip ratio.

KNOW YOUR ENEMY

If you want to stop smoking, it helps to understand just how the addictive substance in tobacco, nicotine, gets a hold on you. When you inhale from a cigarette, a belt of nicotine enters your brain within 10 seconds. That is faster than the entry of almost any other substance, and helps to give nicotine its powerful grip.

Smoking feels good because nicotine is a stimulant. It can make you feel calmer, more energized and more mentally alert. By prompting release of the body's own feel-good chemicals, called endorphins, it can give you a mood boost and lift depression.

These effects are only temporary, however. To sustain them, you need regular doses of nicotine, and after a while the brain adapts, lowering your natural energy and mood levels. So the consequence is that you need to smoke to feel "normal"—and, when you try to quit, you are hit hard by nicotine-withdrawal symptoms including anxiety, depression, impaired concentration and tiredness.

DEVELOP A STRATEGY

That's why it is so crucial to work out in advance a strategy for achieving your aim. Some people manage to quit "cold turkey"—they just stop smoking, and that's it. This approach can be surprisingly successful, especially if you have the right support.

One helpful tactic is to plan ahead, pick a date on which you will have your last cigarette and set about dismantling your psychological associations with smoking—this will make it easier to deal with when the time comes.

If you decide to choose a stop date in advance, make it a day when you are least likely to be stressed and most able to break familiar habits and routines.

Avoid trying to give it up at Christmas, during intense work periods or at times when you are likely to have heavy domestic or family commitments.

Willpower is your main weapon, but studies suggest that the more support you have—be it from friends, family or professionals—the more likely you are to succeed. It is a good idea to talk to your doctor about the help available in your community. Studies also find that people are more

Trying to quit means having to deal with nicotine-withdrawal symptoms, including anxiety, depression and tiredness.

therapies and medications

Your doctor can prescribe nicotine replacement therapy (NRT) in the form of gum, patches or sprays that help to control cravings. These products are generally available without a perscription. NRT releases nicotine into your bloodstream at much lower doses than a cigarette, without the tar, carbon monoxide or other poisonous chemicals you get from tobacco smoke. Most people stop using NRT within three months, but heavy smokers may need to use it for longer.

Your doctor can also perscribe medications to help you quit. These include Zyban (bupropion) and Chantix/Champix (varenicline). Zyban is an antidepressant that affects brain chemicals. It relieves withdrawal symptoms and may double your chances of quitting when used with a counseling program. Varenicline appears to have a better success rate and fewer side effects. It acts on nicotine receptors in the brain, reducing nicotine cravings and lessening the pull of smoking. It, too, is usually taken together with a program. In one study, four weeks after starting treatment, 63 percent of users of Chantix/Champix were still not smoking, compared with 48 percent of those on nicotine replacement therapies and 51 percent of people who quit cold turkey.

likely to be successful at quitting if they work with their health care team. Your doctor can provide individual counseling and refer you to a smoking cessation program. Success rates for people who are aiming to quit are substantially improved by programs that offer support, education, coping skills, counseling and behavior therapy—virtually anything that means the smoker is not left to do it alone. Having the support of your family and friends, too, can make all the difference (see Resources, page 240).

FORWARD PLANNING

Expect the first three days of withdrawal to be the worst, and make plans to ensure that this time is as stress-free but busy as possible—fill it with activities that you find absorbing and calming. If possible, get out of your usual environment. You could book a three-day activity break over a long weekend, take that long-awaited trip to a health spa, join a gym or attend a course that precludes smoking during the day.

If you stay at home, plan to do something outside your usual routine that has a clear goal and visibly positive results: Decorate or do spring cleaning, tackle the garden or do a DIY project. Or simply spend time having long naps, soaking in the bath, reading, listening to music or however else you like to relax.

SUPPORT FROM FAMILY AND FRIENDS

Telling your friends, family and colleagues that you plan to stop smoking makes it far more difficult for you to find excuses to put it off and start "tomorrow" or "next week." Ask those around you to give you their support, encouragement and understanding.

PREPARE YOURSELF

Getting to the bottom of what motivates you to smoke is often important in preparing yourself mentally for giving it up. For example, do you use smoking as an excuse for taking a break from work, as an opportunity to sit down and relax for 5 minutes, to combat stress, tension, tiredness or boredom, or as a substitute for a snack? Do you have a cigarette at social events, when you're under pressure at work or because other people around you are smoking?

Think about what motivators could help you to quit—such as being able to wake up in the morning without coughing, protecting your family from secondhand smoke, avoiding cold winter mornings smoking on the sidewalk outside work or the money you'll save. If you've tried to stop before and gone back to the habit, don't think of that as a failure; think of it as a trial run. However long you stopped on that occasion, it was a success, and now's the time to build on it.

SECRETweapon

BE POSITIVE

Setting a positive goal is much more likely to succeed than focusing on self-denial. Don't tell yourself "I want to quit" or "I shouldn't have a cigarette" (which just draws attention to how much you want one). Think, "I want clearer lungs," "I want to taste my food properly again" or "I want to stay healthy when I get older."

Change your routine—if you are in the habit of having a cigarette with breakfast at home, go to a café instead.

UNLEARN BAD HABITS

Smoking is not just a physical addiction; it is also a learned behaviour and to free yourself from it, you need to unlearn the habits associated with it as well as break the physical addiction. The more you understand how your habit took hold, the greater your chance of breaking it. If you smoke a pack of cigarettes daily, then in the course of a year you take more than 70,000 puffs, each one giving you a temporary "high" as the nicotine hits your brain. But your brain links the high not only with nicotine but also with all the associated gestures you make—the way you take the cigarette out of the pack, and light, inhale and hold it—and with all the situations in which you typically smoke: after a meal, with your morning coffee, after sex, on the phone, when you're working, with a drink.

A long time before the date on which you intend to quit, make a mental list of the situations in which you usually smoke, so that during your first three days you can avoid as far as possible your most common cigarette cues. Start to break the habits, preferably by substituting new ones that give you similar relief and are better for your health.

STOP-SMOKING DAY

When you do stop smoking, take it one day at a time. Simply concentrate on steering clear of cigarettes for that particular day. Your mind can handle thinking "none today," but could start dreaming up reasons for relapsing if you feed it the thought of "no more, ever again."

CONQUER CRAVINGS

The average craving lasts just 3 minutes, though it can seem like hours. Here are some tactics that can help prevent you from caving in:

● **Change your routine** If you usually have a cigarette at the end of a meal, try clearing the plates immediately after you have finished eating, brushing your teeth or making tea. If you typically smoke while you're on the phone, keep some sugar-free gum or mints next to the phone (or with your cell) and chew or suck as you chat. If you usually light up with your morning coffee, switch to tea or fruit juice, or go to a café (non-smoking, of course) for breakfast rather than eating at home.

● **Make it difficult for yourself** Ideally, there should be no cigarettes in the house at all. If you do have some, keep the cigarette pack on the other side of the room, in a cabinet or even a locked drawer. Do not bring cigarettes with you when you go out.

● **Relieve work stress** Instead of joining the smoking-break huddle on the sidewalk outside your office, go for a quick stroll around the block. It will improve your mood and relieve feelings of tension.

● **Distract yourself** Train your brain to unlearn the expectation of an instant nicotine reward. When you think you want a cigarette, persuade yourself to wait 5 minutes, then 10. When you want to give in, find something—anything—to do to take your mind off cigarettes. Take a shower, pull up a few weeds, brush your teeth or take out the garbage.

DEFENSEtactics

WHAT TO DRINK

For the first three days after quitting, sip acidic fruit juices such as cranberry, grapefruit or pineapple. They can help to stabilize blood-sugar levels and accelerate elimination of nicotine during the crucial first 72 hours.

Be careful with alcohol, though. Almost half of those who relapse while trying to quit smoking do it after drinking. Alcohol reduces inhibitions and speeds up the metabolism of nicotine, so it can exacerbate withdrawal symptoms and make you more likely to give in—especially as people typically smoke when they're drinking. It makes sense to avoid alcohol for 72 hours.

Nicotine doubles the rate at which caffeine is metabolized, so your blood caffeine levels can more than double if you drink the same amount of coffee or tea as you did prior to quitting. As this can increase feelings of anxiety and make quitting even harder, it's smart to avoid caffeine or at least cut back on your intake.

countdown to good health

Some of the health benefits of quitting smoking take place fairly quickly. Here is what happens to your body during those first smoke-free days and afterwards. The benefits are similar whether you take the cold-turkey approach or use nicotine-replacement products.

Time since stopping	Health improvement
8 hours	The carbon monoxide levels in your blood reduce by half and oxygen levels increase, returning to normal. Circulation improves, so your hands and feet get warmer.
24 hours	Carbon monoxide is eliminated from the body.
48 hours	Your ability to taste and smell improve.
72 hours	Breathing ability (lung function) begins to improve.
14 days	Blood circulation in the gums is virtually back to normal.
1 month	Skin appearance improves.
1 to 3 months	Lung function and breathing improve, so walking and other exercises become easier.
1 year	The risk of heart attack reduces by up to 50 percent compared to that of a smoker.
5 years	Your risk of dying prematurely from heart disease or stroke is now almost equal to that of someone who has never smoked.

● **Don't go without breakfast** When you are a smoker, you can often get away with having no breakfast. When you give up smoking, missing breakfast can make you much more susceptible to a cigarette craving or snacking on too many of the wrong foods later in the day.

INSTANT BENEFITS

The great thing about giving up smoking is that, when you do quit, you will feel the benefits almost immediately. After just 24 smoke-free hours, the supply of oxygen to your heart muscle begins to improve. After one to three months, you will find that you can exercise more freely.

If you've already had a heart attack, quitting smoking will halve your risk of having another one, and reduce your risk of dying from a further attack by a quarter. Within five years, your risk drops almost to that of a someone who has never smoked and your added risk of stroke virtually disappears, no matter how old you are.

BODY DETOX

For every two hours that you get by without smoking, your body's nicotine reserves reduce by half. That sounds good—but it takes up to 72 hours before your blood, and therefore your brain, is completely free of nicotine. It is at this point, three days after your last puff, that the cravings, tension and anxiety associated with quitting typically reach their peak.

The average smoker experiences six cravings on the third day after giving up. That is just 18 minutes in total on the very worst day. Knowing this can help to put those urges in perspective. If you can hold on till the end of three smoke-free days, you've made it through the chemical withdrawal symptoms and are on your way to stopping for good. But remember that a single drag on a cigarette can stimulate up to half of all the brain receptors linked with nicotine addiction. So don't give in even once!

MYTHS

PUTTING ON WEIGHT IS AS BAD FOR YOUR HEALTH AS SMOKING

This is true only if you gain a vast amount of weight. You would need to put on around 75 lb to expose yourself to the same level of risk as smoking a pack of cigarettes a day—and fewer than 4 percent of smokers gain more than 20 lb. In fact, the average weight gain among people who stop smoking is about 5 lb, and about one in five people who stop smoking don't put on weight at all.

AVOID WEIGHT GAIN

Smokers tend to put on a little weight when they give it up, perhaps because of a change in metabolism, or perhaps because they are eating more or eating high-fat and sugary foods to compensate for not smoking. The body may be adjusting to what should be its "normal" weight (smokers tend to weigh less than non-smokers). In addition, recovering smokers are more likely to react to hunger cues by binge eating, because their brains are used to the "quick fix" of nicotine. Here are some tips on how to avoid weight gain:

- Anticipate hunger—avoid binge eating and carbohydrate cravings by eating frequently and choosing small amounts of healthy foods.
- Plan your meals and don't buy sugary or fatty snacks.
- Don't use candy to help you quit smoking—if you need something to satisfy oral cravings, try sugar-free gum.
- If you are tempted to satisfy a nicotine craving with a calorie-laden snack, take a couple of deep breaths or sip a glass of cold water instead. Strangely, our brains sometimes confuse hunger and thirst, so we may think we are hungry when, in fact, we need something to drink.
- Step up your activity levels—walk a little bit farther or a little bit faster, or use the stairs instead of the elevator.

Exposure to cold temperatures places a strain on the heart and cardiovascular system.

no.4 cold weather

Cold weather is something you cannot escape unless you are fortunate enough to live in an area with a mild climate. Older people are particularly vulnerable to cold—partly because they may be less able to detect a drop in temperature, and partly because many of them cannot afford to heat their homes effectively. Exposure to cold temperatures puts a strain on the heart and cardiovascular system. In response, our blood vessels tend to constrict, increasing blood pressure as well as making blood more likely to clot. At the same time, the body's demand for oxygen increases to try to maintain body temperature, so supplies to vital organs such as the heart may be insufficient.

This helps to explain why there are more deaths from heart disease in December and January than in June and July. Other heart problems, such as heart failure (where the heart isn't pumping strongly enough), also peak in winter.

Ideally, try to keep your house heated to between 64° and 70°F (18° and 21°C) in the winter, and remember to dress in warm clothes. Keeping active and eating a healthy diet will also help to protect you.

AVOID EXTREMES

Avoid sudden changes in temperature. Going from a warm, centrally heated house out into the cold without being properly insulated can be especially dangerous. So, too, can a sudden increased level of exertion—especially because people tend to exercise less during the colder months, so their general level of fitness may be reduced. If you really have to go outside to clear snow from your driveway in the morning—the peak time for heart attacks—do the minimum necessary, dress warmly and go slowly.

STOP COMFORT EATING

Another factor in winter-related deaths may be that blood becomes more concentrated in cold weather, so cholesterol levels rise more in autumn and winter than spring and summer. Avoid eating larger quantities than usual in winter, especially more carbohydrate-rich "comfort foods." These dietary changes could contribute to raising cholesterol levels as well as promoting weight gain and metabolic changes. Instead, choose homemade soups, baked apples, clementines and other healthy alternatives.

no.5 respiratory infections

While the common cold may not do much harm, a severe infection such as flu, bronchitis or pneumonia more than doubles the risk of a heart attack or stroke, according to an analysis of medical records of more than 2 million patients published in the *European Heart Journal*. Respiratory infections cause a body-wide inflammatory response that affects blood vessels and can precipitate rupture of plaque in artery walls.

For this reason, doctors recommend that people with heart disease have an annual flu vaccination. Even if it doesn't stop you from getting the infection, it may make it less severe and reduce complications.

BACTERIAL CONNECTIONS

Scientists believe that low-grade infection may be implicated not only in atherosclerosis, but also in a host of other conditions, such as diabetes and even some cancers. Evidence is also growing that infections may be an important trigger for age-related diseases and disorders. One team of Russian doctors has even suggested that infection may be what initiates the very process of aging. Along with many specific diseases, aging itself, they say, "has infectious origins." This indicates that safeguarding yourself from mild infections such as flu or gum disease may protect you not only against heart attacks, strokes and an early demise, but also against many of the other conditions underlying the infirmity and disability that often accompany old age.

HOW GERMS ARE SPREAD

You may have heard the old saying: "Coughs and sneezes spread diseases." That statement is perfectly true, but what it doesn't tell you is that colds and flu are far more often spread by other means, such as shaking hands, turning a door handle or picking up a telephone that's been used by someone else.

It is actually quite difficult to catch a cold. Close-range coughing or sneezing can spread an infection, but the spread is much more likely to occur through contact with contaminated fingers—shaking someone's hand is potentially more risky than kissing them. Recent research has shown that respiratory viruses can lurk on hard surfaces for up to two days. What typically happens is that you shake someone's hand, then rub your nose or eyes—something that most people do unconsciously all the time. If the person whose hand you shook has a cold, you may well be infected too. Touching your eyes can introduce infection because the tear ducts drain into the back of the nose.

WASH YOUR HANDS ...

The key to protecting yourself is as simple as washing your hands regularly and thoroughly. So avoid a vigorous handshake whenever you can, and go for a vigorous hand-wash instead. In fact, frequent hand-washing has been shown to reduce the transmission of colds even between members of the same household.

... AND SURFACES

Another effective way to ward off colds and flu is regular disinfection of household surfaces—ordinary diluted bleach will do. Door handles, taps or faucets and refrigerator doors are particular culprits for transmitting infection, and telephones, computer keyboards, light switches, kitchen surfaces and cleaning cloths may also harbor germs.

For situations where you can't avoid contact with other people's germs, carry a small bottle of alcohol-based sanitizing hand gel or spray with you and use it after shaking hands or touching public surfaces.

COLD CONTAMINATION

One study assessed how easily cold viruses could be transferred from ordinary surfaces to fingertips. Researchers asked 15 adults with colds caused by rhinoviruses (which cause about half of all colds) to stay overnight in a hotel, then tested ten hard surfaces in each room. Of the total 150 sites tested, 35 percent were contaminated with cold viruses. The most contaminated surfaces were door handles, pens, light switches, television remote controls, faucets and telephones.

The researchers then asked five volunteers to touch the light switches, telephone keypads or handsets and tested their fingertips for rhinoviruses. When the tests were made an hour after contamination, the subjects' fingertips had become contaminated 60 percent of the time. Even 18 hours later, contamination was found in a third of the tests. The researchers concluded that people with colds frequently contaminate surfaces in their environment, and that cold viruses can then be picked up by others during the course of normal daily activities.

The problem with trying to ward off cold viruses is that, when you are out in public, you have no idea which surfaces have been touched by someone with a virus. What's worse, most respiratory infections are caught

beat off those germs

- **Go Gallic** The evidence that hands are a major route for transmitting infection is so strong that scientists at the London School of Hygiene in the United Kingdom recommend greeting friends the French way: with a peck on the cheek rather than a handshake. Or improvise according to the situation. The next time someone approaches you with palm outstretched, try an "air kiss" or manly hug instead.
- **Disinfect household surfaces regularly** Door handles, taps, television remote controls and refrigerator doors may all be repositories for germs. Other culprits include telephones, computer keyboards, light switches, kitchen surfaces and cleaning cloths.
- **Use your microwave** Keep your kitchen sponge or cloth germ-free by microwaving it on full power for 2 minutes daily. This kills 99 percent of microorganisms. **WARNING:** Do this only with a damp sponge or cloth—otherwise it might catch on fire.
- **Take a walk** One study showed that postmenopausal women who did regular, moderate exercise—brisk walking for 45 minutes, five times a week—had up to a three-fold reduction in the number of colds they suffered, compared with women who didn't exercise.
- **Say cheers** Scientists in Spain have shown that wine, especially red wine, also protects against colds. When they studied 4,000 volunteers for a year, they found that those who drank more than two glasses of red wine daily had 44 percent fewer colds than non-drinkers.
- **Take garlic** In a study involving 146 volunteers, half were given a garlic supplement daily and the other half a placebo. During 90 days over the winter, those taking garlic had a total of 24 colds between them, compared with 65 among those on placebo. People taking garlic supplements who did get sick also got better faster, and had a lower risk of reinfection.
- **Bolster immunity** A healthy diet with a generous intake of fruit and vegetables, exercise and seven hours of sleep daily can all make your body less vulnerable to germs.

from close contact with someone in your home, especially a school-age child. Surfaces are readily contaminated too, so when one person—or a visitor—is carrying a virus, everyone in the household is at risk.

HOW TO AVOID COLDS AND FLU

Research confirms that hand-washing and frequent disinfection of surfaces are the most effective ways to protect yourself against colds and flu.

When researchers ran a campaign promoting hand-washing and giving out hand-sanitizer gel among students in university dorms, they found that these students had fewer episodes of colds and flu and missed fewer classes as a result, compared with students who were not part of the campaign. And, according to a Canadian study, using a disinfectant spray on a surface contaminated by cold viruses reduced the virus counts by more than 99.99 percent in just 1 minute.

no.6 lack of sunshine

Regular exposure to sunlight is essential for good health. Sunlight on skin prompts our bodies to make vitamin D, which may help to protect against heart disease, high blood pressure, strokes and many cancers, as well as warding off disorders such as diabetes and rheumatoid arthritis.

Studies conducted in the UK concluded that frequently gray skies could contribute to heart attack and stroke levels by depleting people's vitamin D. A North American study found that those with low vitamin-D levels ran a 62 percent higher risk of heart attack or stroke. Low levels of the vitamin have been linked with increased rates of cardiovascular disease, more colds, flu and other diseases. One ten-year study of 18,000 men aged 40 to 75, who were initially free of cardiovascular disease, indicated that low vitamin-D levels more than doubled their risk of heart attacks and coronary artery disease.

NOT GETTING ENOUGH?

As we have seen, our bodies make the majority of our vitamin D from the ultraviolet light that hits our skin, specifically UVB rays. But we have a predilection to slather on sunscreen and this, coupled with the lack of sunlight during the winter months and in northern climates, prompts experts to warn that we are facing an "epidemic" of vitamin-D deficiency, with darker-skinned people and all individuals over 50 running the greatest risk.

In winter, it's worth trying to increase your intake of foods that contain vitamin D, such as milk.

VITAMIN D IN FOODS

Although most of the vitamin D present in our bodies is made by sunlight, small amounts can be obtained from foods such as oily fish. So, especially in the winter, try to increase your intake of foods that contain vitamin D. As well as oily fish like salmon, fresh tuna, sardines and herring, good sources of vitamin D include cod liver oil, eggs, dairy products like milk and cheese, and fortified foods such as breakfast cereals and margarines.

Just 15 to 20 minutes with your arms, hands and legs exposed will keep your vitamin D at adequate levels.

THE VALUE OF SUPPLEMENTS

Taking vitamin D supplements can have a beneficial effect on your health. Research studies indicate that supplements reduce levels of inflammation, which is believed to be closely associated with heart disease (see page 22), and that a combination of vitamin D and calcium supplements can lower high blood pressure.

One study demonstrated that people who took vitamin D supplements had 70 percent fewer episodes of colds and flu over three years—and, as explained earlier, respiratory infections have also been linked with an increased risk of cardiovascular disease. Other research has indicated a 31 percent lower death rate from heart disease among women over 65 who took vitamin D supplements, while a European review of 18 studies found that taking supplements for six years reduced the death rate from all causes by 7 percent.

If you decide to take supplements, most experts recommend taking at least 1,000 IU (25 mcg) a day. If you suffer from a vitamin-D deficiency, your doctor may recommend much higher doses—but don't take more than 1000 IU of vitamin D a day without talking to your doctor first.

GET OUT IN THE SUN

You can't overdose on vitamin D from the sun, and that is the best source. More than 90 percent of the vitamin D in our bodies is made in our skin when it is exposed to the ultraviolet light in the sun's rays. Once our skin has absorbed enough UVB rays to make vitamin D, the conversion process shuts down.

Not much is needed to achieve the desired effect. As little as 15 to 20 minutes daily with your arms, hands and legs exposed will keep your vitamin D at adequate levels. That is why some doctors now recommend spending 15 minutes toward midday outdoors without sunscreen (except on your face), several times a week—unless your skin is very fair and burns during even brief exposure. If you are black, Asian or South Asian, your skin might not be as efficient at absorbing the UVB rays that trigger vitamin D production, and you may need twice the time in the sun.

If the recommended time is up and you plan to be out longer, put on plenty of sunscreen to protect yourself against the sun damage that can lead to skin cancers.

By getting enough vitamin D from the sun in the spring, summer and autumn, you will enter the first weeks of winter in good form. But from then on, you must rely on diet (and perhaps a daily supplement) until spring—and sunlight—return.

no.7 extreme heat

Very hot summers have been shown to provoke a small increase in death rates, mainly from cardiovascular and respiratory diseases. While extreme heat is not as dangerous as extreme cold—tens of thousands of mainly older people die from cold-related causes every winter, compared with hundreds of deaths during the worst heat waves—it still makes sense to protect yourself against it.

Older people are most vulnerable to heatstroke, but younger people can also succumb. Women are affected more often than men. In one study in London in the UK, for every 1.8°F (1°C) rise in temperature above 68°F (20°C), mortality rates increased by an average of 3 percent in men and 7 percent in women aged between 75 and 84. People living in cities are

People in cities are especially at risk of heat-related health problems, since roads and buildings contain and reflect heat.

especially at risk of heat-related health problems, since roads and buildings contain and reflect heat, creating "heat islands" with temperatures several degrees above those of surrounding areas.

If your home is in a town or city, it is probably unrealistic to consider moving to the countryside. But wherever you are, it is advisable to take precautions. Since around a third of the deaths that occur as a result of extreme heat waves are thought to be caused by air pollution (see pages 196–97), it is also worth taking measures to limit your exposure to traffic and other noxious fumes.

WHAT YOU CAN DO

In hot weather, stay indoors during the part of the day when temperatures are highest, and close the curtains on windows that get full sun. When outside, wear a broad-brimmed hat with light-colored, loose clothing and stay in the shade as much as you can. Make use of electric fans if available. If you are out in extreme heat, try to go to places with air conditioning, even if this involves no more than a stroll around your local mall. Make sure that you drink enough fluid to prevent dehydration. You can tell whether you're drinking enough by the color of your urine: It should be a pale straw color at most, but if it is any darker, you need to drink more.

no.8 air pollution

People who live in heavily polluted areas have a higher-than-average risk of developing cardiovascular disease, and smog can worsen symptoms in people with heart and circulatory disease—hospital admissions among patients with heart disease increase during periods of high air pollution.

Pollution raises blood pressure and can trigger heart attacks and strokes, especially in people who are already vulnerable. Exhaust fumes are a major contaminating factor, say epidemiologists; studies suggest they can adversely affect arteries and reduce oxygen supply to the heart.

WHAT'S IN THE AIR?

It's the minute particles in polluted air, generated by vehicles, factories and electricity generators, which seem to do the most damage. These can penetrate deep into the lungs, causing inflammation. A high proportion is retained in the lungs, and a tiny amount gets absorbed into the body.

Air pollution causes blood vessels to narrow, even in healthy people, which may explain why high pollution levels increase the rate of heart attacks and other cardiovascular problems in people with cardiovascular disease. Researchers found that after breathing air polluted with fine particles and ozone for just two hours, the blood vessels of 25 healthy volunteers narrowed by between 2 and 4 percent.

Being exposed to diesel exhaust fumes reduces the amount of oxygen that reaches the heart during exercise. When a group of men who had recovered from a heart attack exercised for an hour in a room polluted with low levels of diesel fumes, tests revealed a three-fold leap in the amount of stress on the heart—enough to increase the risk of a heart attack. The concentration of diesel fumes in the room was kept to just 10 percent of the typical pollution levels in city centers, suggesting that real-life exercise in urban environments may be even more hazardous.

People who live in cities with clean-air policies may add an extra five months to their lifespan, compared with those living in more polluted places. One study found that those who had more exposure to traffic-related pollution were 20 percent more likely to die at any time than those with less exposure, and 40 percent more likely to die from heart disease.

Doctors frequently recommend that people recovering from a heart attack should not drive in heavy traffic for a few weeks because of the stress this creates—which is another reason for everyone to avoid heavy traffic congestion whenever possible.

It's important not to stop exercising, so head for the park.

CHECK THE FORECAST

It is not always possible to avoid air pollution, but you can take steps to reduce your exposure. You can check your local air quality-pollution index along with daily weather forecasts. In the car, drive with your windows closed on major roads or downtown, especially on smoggy days. If you can, plan a route away from heavily congested areas.

EXERCISE CAUTION

You are especially at risk from the effects of pollution when doing exercise because you breathe more often and more deeply, inhaling more pollutants and sucking them further down into your lungs. Athletes also tend to breathe through the mouth more than normal, bypassing the effective filters against particles provided by hair and mucus in the nose. So, when possible, try to breathe through your nose.

It is important not to abandon exercise, but try to avoid the rush hour, or exercise in green open spaces away from heavy traffic, especially on days when the pollution index is high. Keep away from roads and, whenever possible, walk, run or cycle in a park or the countryside.

troubleshooting Q&A

I live near a cell-phone tower. Does this increase my risk of having a heart attack?

Probably not. Repeated studies have shown no effect on health of exposure to low-level radio-frequency energies—in terms either of overall well-being or of cardiovascular health.

no.9 noise

There is another reason, apart from pollution, to avoid heavy traffic: The sheer noise may be dangerous. Living with chronic noise exposure increases the risk of heart attacks, and the World Health Organization (WHO) warns that long-term noise exposure above 67 to 70 dB (equivalent to traffic noise) can lead to high blood pressure. When researchers assessed people who had been admitted to 32 major hospitals in Berlin following a heart attack, they found that environmental noise increased risk more than three-fold in women, and by 45 percent in men. Overall, people living in high-traffic areas were 46 percent more at risk than those living in quieter areas.

Theories about why noise can do physical harm include its association with increased stress and irritation, leading to an outpouring of stress hormones and rises in heart rate, blood pressure and blood lipids. People who already have cardiovascular disease may be at special risk, and noise can provoke changes in heart rhythm.

PROTECT YOUR HEARING

If your work involves loud noise, it is sensible to wear noise-canceling earplugs at all times as recommended by your employer. Similarly, make sure that you protect your ears if you engage in noisy sports like shooting.

But the harm may start at low levels, and there are countless noisy tasks in daily life that we may do without thinking of the potential damage to our cardiovascular system (or our hearing).

So buy several pairs of good-quality earplugs with a high noise-reduction rating (NRR) and use them whenever you undertake noisy tasks such as mowing the lawn or using power tools.

Small specialized earplugs, called flat-attenuation or flat-response earplugs, are available for use at events like rock concerts; when using them, you are still able to hear the music clearly, but they protect you from hazardous amplified noise levels.

REDalert **!**

SLEEPING WITH THE ENEMY

If your partner is a snorer, chances are you're subjected to noise levels overnight sufficient to disturb your sleep and raise your risk of cardiovascular disease. A loud snorer can emit sounds of up to 95 dB—equal to a heavy truck thundering past at close range. One study showed increases in blood pressure among people sleeping with snorers. In addition, snorers are themselves at high risk of cardiovascular disease.

The best way to resolve this problem is to persuade your partner to see his or her doctor for tests, assessment and treatment. Meanwhile, get yourself some special snore-attenuating earplugs (visit the American Sleep Apnea Association at sleepapnea.org or the Canadian Sleep Society at css.to for more information).

If your work involves loud noise, take care to protect your ears at all times.

is it **too loud?**

How can you tell if the sounds in your life have the potential to harm your hearing and cardiovascular health? Damage may be occurring if:

- You are exposed to regular heavy-impact noises such as pneumatic drills and hammering.
- You use heavy power tools for more than 30 minutes a day.
- You are exposed to continuous noise at work during the day—in an airport, on a building site or in a factory that has loud industrial machinery or power tools—or in the evening at a nightclub.
- You experience ringing in your ears (tinnitus) during or after noise exposure.

Hearing impairment can also be caused by prolonged exposure to the noise of a motorcycle engine (90–100 dB), a loud car stereo (95–140 dB) or even the inside of a busy bar (90–95 dB).

TURN IT DOWN

If you are exposed to loud background noise for long periods, try to reduce the noise level or minimize your exposure to it, and minimize noise at other times. Studies find that chronic noise exposure increases blood pressure which, in turn, increases the risk of heart disease and stroke.

NIGHTTIME NOISE

Chronic nighttime noise above 50 dB—the level of light traffic—poses a risk to cardiovascular health, says the WHO. Other studies suggest that traffic noise above 30 dB may cause you to lose sleep, a hazard in itself. The fact is that many people these days live in noisy cities, sometimes with enough nighttime noise to disrupt their sleep.

If you get traffic noise in your home, hang heavy curtains and consider double-glazing your windows. If it's still noisy at night, try using earplugs or a white-noise machine to help you sleep.

no.10 toxic chemicals

Chemicals in the environment may be implicated in a variety of medical conditions that have become more common in the past century, including cancer, allergies, asthma, skin disease, autoimmune conditions such as rheumatoid arthritis and multiple sclerosis, and cardiovascular disease.

Heavy metals such as lead, mercury and cadmium are known to be linked to the risk of heart disease and strokes. In fact, some experts recommend that anyone who has high blood pressure, heart disease or another vascular disease should be tested for heavy metal toxicity.

- Lead is widespread, and long-term, low-level exposure has been linked with atherosclerosis, thrombosis (blood clots), high blood pressure and cardiovascular disease. If you live in an old house, make sure that the pipes are not made of lead, which could leach into the water supply. And be careful when redecorating—old paints often contain lead.
- Mercury increases inflammation, promotes clotting and damages the function of arterial linings. Mercury toxicity can cause high blood pressure and cardiovascular disease, and increases the risk of strokes and heart attacks. Pregnant women should avoid eating certain types of fish that may be contaminated with high levels of mercury (see page 106). Taking selenium supplements may help to reduce its toxicity.
- Cadmium, used industrially in metal alloys, can cause kidney damage and lead to high blood pressure, blood sugar and body fat imbalances, and zinc deficiency. Eating calcium-rich foods can reduce its toxic effects.
- Iron can promote atherosclerosis, so cutting back on iron-rich foods such as red meat may be a good idea. In one study of people who had already had a heart attack or stroke, limiting iron intake seemed to reduce the risk of a second attack. But a reasonable intake of iron is required for vital body functions and to prevent anemia, so talk to your doctor before making any major changes to your diet.

PLASTIC PACKAGING ALERT

British researchers have found that people with a high level of the chemical bisphenol A (BPA) in their urine are twice as likely to develop cardiovascular disease and diabetes—findings that back up BPA studies conducted elsewhere.

BPA is a phthalate, one of a family of chemical compounds used as plasticizers, mainly to increase the flexibility of PVC and other plastic products. BPA was widely present in hard plastic packaging used for food and drink containers, including water bottles, plastic (polycarbonate) baby' bottles and the linings of food cans. Many companies now also produce BPA-free versions of their products.

In 2010, the US Environmental Protection Agency released a report calling BPA a chemical of concern, while the President's Cancer Panel called for caution pertaining to BPA. Canada was the first country to ban the sale of baby bottles containing BPA in 2008, and listed it as a toxic substance in 2010. Some US states have passed or are exploring similar bans.

PHTHALATES ARE EVERYWHERE

Even with less BPA in food and drink containers, it is still nearly impossible to avoid some exposure to phthalates. For example, many foods are sold in plastic packaging (it may be wise to remove it soon after purchase). Phthalates may be present in cosmetics, shampoos, adhesives, detergents and paints. As the kind of paint used on the outside of ships usually includes phthalates, the chemicals are increasingly present in fish. BPA is also found in drinking water and on skin—and consequently in household dust (largely derived from shed skin cells). Researchers find that more than 93 percent of Americans and 91 percent of Canadians have detectable levels of BPA.

CARDIOVASCULAR LINK

Evidence linking obesity with phthalates and other so-called "endocrine-disrupting" chemicals is growing—so much so, that many of these substances are now dubbed "obesogens," or obesity-promoting chemicals.

Clearly, their association with obesity is one mechanism by which chemicals such as BPA could influence the development of cardiovascular disease, and some studies have demonstrated links between phthalate breakdown products in urine and BMI, waist circumference (a measure of abdominal obesity) and insulin resistance.

ten times safer

Sensible caution and finding ways to break the grip of any potentially harmful addictions are the best responses to the physical hazards outlined here, and the strategies suggested will help you to combat them effectively.

Your self-defense plan is almost complete. But as you'll discover, after physical hazards, there are still mental barriers. Step 9 outlines the psychological factors which also influence your cardiovascular health.

self-defense plan

STEP

9

CONTENTMENT, A SENSE OF HUMOR, **HAPPY RELATIONSHIPS AND** STIMULATING INTERESTS WILL ALL HELP TO PROTECT YOU AGAINST CARDIOVASCULAR PROBLEMS. STRESS, ANGER AND DEPRESSION, **HOWEVER, CAN RAISE BLOOD PRESSURE AND ACCELERATE** THE PROGRESSION OF ATHEROSCLEROSIS. BUT THERE ARE TACTICS YOU CAN **ADOPT TO COUNTER THE** NEGATIVE ELEMENTS OF LIFE AND PUT YOU BACK IN CONTROL.

Relax and enjoy life

Nothing can have a greater impact on your well-being than the way you look after yourself – and one of the best ways to maintain both physical and mental health is to act and think positively. Calm resistance to the adverse influences of stress, hostility and hopelessness can work wonders in the fight against heart attacks and strokes. And, as you will see, friendship, laughter and an outgoing, optimistic attitude are the golden tickets to a longer life.

taking stress seriously

Stress is one of the most significant indirect causes of illness in the modern world and plays a key part in triggering cardiovascular emergencies. It is one of the nine factors that, according to the Interheart study (see page 17), underlies 90 percent of all first heart attacks. Recent research has revealed that, if you are permanently stressed at work or at home, you double your risk of a heart attack. Factors carrying the highest risk include a major conflict between family members and intense financial pressures, such as business failure. Stress is also a significant risk factor for stroke.

THE EFFECTS OF STRESS

When we feel that an event or situation is stressful, our bodies' learned defense mechanism against danger—the "fight or flight" response—kicks in. This leads to an increased release of adrenaline and other stress hormones, causing the heart to beat stronger and faster, raising our blood pressure and breathing rate, promoting sweating (because the body anticipates intense activity, and sweat helps to regulate body temperature) and shutting down digestion and other non-essential functions. This response would have been helpful in the Stone Age, when we might have confronted by wild animals;

it is much less so in the face of irritating, automated telephone help lines and traffic jams. Persistent stress can lead to high blood pressure and a raised clotting tendency—a risk factor for both heart attacks and strokes. Stress also prompts the body to release a hormone called cortisol, long-term exposure to which has been linked with abdominal obesity, high blood pressure and Type 2 diabetes.

A sudden rise in blood pressure, stimulated by acute stress, can also cause hemorrhagic strokes (bleeding in the brain). Stress increases your risk of strokes by as much as 40 percent.

People under stress are more likely to smoke, drink, eat unhealthily, get less exercise and find it hard to sleep.

OFFICE OFFENSIVE

North Americans work some of the longest hours in the world, and many of us admit that work stress spills over into our private lives, making us grumpy at home. Medical research links stress at work to an increased cardiovascular risk. In 2008, when British scientists analyzed data from a 12-year study of 10,000 civil servants, they found that men and women under 50 who reported long-term work stress had a 68 percent increased risk of coronary artery disease. The risk was lower among those at retirement age. Those reporting the highest levels of work stress had high morning levels of the stress hormone cortisol and a consistently raised heart rate—evidence of increased cardiac instability.

Dealing with an unfair boss can send your blood pressure soaring. In one study, researchers measured the blood pressure of female health-care assistants over three working days. When some of the women worked under a supervisor they perceived as unfair, they showed average increases in systolic blood pressure (the top reading) of 15mmHg, and in diastolic pressure (the bottom reading) of 7mmHg—more than enough to produce a significant increase in the risk of both heart attacks and strokes. Having a boss you consider incompetent raises your risk, too.

I'm under a great deal of pressure right now. Am I at risk of having a heart attack or stroke?

Pressure or stress can have a detrimental effect on your health, but it is all a question of how you handle it. You may not be able to avoid pressure, but you can learn ways to cope with it—and some people actually thrive under pressure. If your stress is making you tense or miserable or interfering with your sleep—or if you react by smoking, eating high-fat sugary foods or drinking more alcohol—then your unhealthy habits are putting you at increased risk of a heart attack or stroke. Changing your lifestyle can help you to feel healthier and better able to cope with these demands, and there are plenty of things you can do to help you relax and manage stress.

EASING THE TENSION

If your manager's behavior makes your blood boil, it is important to learn ways of handling your frustration (see page 210). Try not to tense up in a difficult situation. Standing straight, with a relaxed posture, will give you more confidence and control. If you do have a confrontation, get away from the scene of the conflict as soon as you can. Even if it's just for 5 minutes, go for a walk and give yourself a chance to breathe, loosen up and clear your mind.

While you may not be able to affect your levels of cortisol in the mornings, you can make a substantial difference to other lifestyle factors that increase your risk. Researchers find that people under stress smoke more, eat fewer fruits and vegetables, and exercise less. They are also more likely to have components of metabolic syndrome, all of which helps explain why work stress can increase the risk of heart disease by nearly a third. So if your work is piling on the pressure, don't pile on the pounds or engage in other unhealthy coping strategies. Pay attention to your diet and stay active. And remember that exercise will help to relieve stress and anxiety.

REDalert **!**

DEADLINE DANGER

Meeting a demanding work deadline can make some people more susceptible to heart attack over the following 24 hours. Swedish researchers assessed 1,381 men and women who had survived a heart attack and asked them about their work in the previous year.

It turned out that 8 percent of the group—almost one in ten—had faced a high-pressure deadline at work in the 24 hours before their attack, and that such pressure was linked to a staggering sixfold increase in heart-attack risk over the following day. This short-term pressure was far more dangerous than an accumulation of less stressful events over the previous year.

Try to manage tight deadlines by planning ahead. If your workload is unmanageable, talk to your manager or your human resources team—that's what they're there for.

WEEKDAY BLUES

Stress levels are at their highest on Monday mornings—also the peak time for strokes, heart attacks and heart-rhythm problems. Heart attacks are around 20 percent more common on Mondays than on other days, among retired people as well as the employed. Just getting ready for work on Monday can cause some people's blood pressure to rise. The prospect of the week ahead is not the only cause: For some, it's the aftereffects of a weekend of heavy drinking, which can cause dangerously abnormal heart rhythms and raise blood pressure (see page 175). For others, it's the pressure of the daily commute.

To improve your commute, travel later or earlier one morning a week if you can to avoid traffic jams. If you can, try biking or walking to work. This is called "active commuting," and studies find that it can significantly reduce the risk of heart disease and stroke.

COPING STRATEGIES

Here are some simple but useful techniques to help you to stay on top of your workload:

- Ask to work flextime so you can commute outside peak hours. (As long as you get the work done, many employers are sympathetic.)
- Cycle or walk part of the way to work. You'll burn up stress hormones and get some exercise.
- Make a to-do list for the day.
- Set realistic goals. Make them clear and achievable.
- Manage your time. Don't try to cram too much into your schedule, and avoid taking on anything else until you've completed the task at hand.
- Break big tasks into small steps.
- Settle for less than perfect. Work at 90 percent of your capacity rather

than 110 percent—and delegate.
- Regulate the time you spend dealing with e-mails. You could set up an automatic e-mail response that reads "I answer e-mails at 10 am, 1 pm and 4 pm. If you need a quick reply, please call me."
- Let your phone switch over to voice mail while you're finishing a task.
- If you spend most of your time sitting at work, do some exercises at your desk (see page 148) to relieve the strain.
- Always stop work during your lunch hour and, preferably, get a change of scenery. Try not to discuss work during the break.
- Learn some rapid stress-relief techniques to use at times of tension (see page 213). Simply closing your eyes for a few moments and clearing your mind can reenergize you during a frenetic day.
- Leave work on time.
- Don't take work home.
- Don't check your work e-mail when you're at home or on vacation.

PERSONAL PROBLEMS

Stressful relationships at home can increase your risk of having a heart attack or stroke by more than a third. Relationships are an important barometer of your happiness. If you can't resolve sensitive family issues, consult a counsellor (see Resources, page 240).

Catastrophic events such as a death or serious illness in the family can cause a surge in stress hormones that temporarily "stun" the heart. Some people develop symptoms such as chest pain and breathlessness that mimic those of a heart attack—and, in some cases, heart failure may occur after a severe emotional trauma. Fortunately, however, any damage to heart muscle is usually reversible.

HOLIDAY ATTACK

Stress is also partly responsible for the rise in heart attacks and strokes during the festive season. There are two noticeable peaks: Christmas and New Year's Day. It's not just overindulgence in fatty foods and alcohol that's to blame. Research indicates that the cause is the emotional stress of the winter holidays: dealing with relatives, too much traveling, not enough sleep, the expenses involved and even cooking holiday dinner.

Continued on p212 ➤

know yourself:
your reaction to stress

Some stress is necessary in our lives; it keeps us motivated and enthusiastic. For example, being under pressure to complete a piece of work on time can boost creativity. But it's important to get the balance right.

Everyone reacts differently to stress. Some people take it in stride; others become tense, angry, irritable or tearful; and some lose concentration or reach for "comfort foods," alcohol or cigarettes. None of these responses are good for you.

When British scientists studied 34 men who had recovered from heart attacks or acute chest pain, they found that 14 had experienced emotional stress—such as an argument with a neighbor or sadness about a sick or deceased relative—less than two hours before their heart attack. The remaining 20 men reported no stress before their heart attacks. All the men were given a series of mentally challenging tests, such as making a speech, to raise stress levels, and they all showed short-term increases in blood pressure and heart rate. But the blood pressure levels of the 14 men who had reported stress, anger or depression just before their heart attack took longer to return to normal. They also had higher levels of platelets in their blood, which increases the chances of dangerous blood clots forming; in the other men, the levels were unchanged.

ARE YOU SUFFERING FROM STRESS? FIND OUT HOW MANY OF THE FOLLOWING SIGNS AND SYMPTOMS APPLY TO YOU:

- ☐ Feeling sweaty or shivery
- ☐ Pounding heart or palpitations
- ☐ Needing to go to the toilet more often than usual
- ☐ Feeling sick in the stomach (having "butterflies")
- ☐ Dry mouth
- ☐ Feeling tired, having no energy
- ☐ Odd aches and pains
- ☐ Smoking more than you used to
- ☐ Drinking more (needing a drink to relax)
- ☐ Working to the point of exhaustion
- ☐ Headaches

- ☐ Disturbed sleep, waking unusually early
- ☐ Being easily irritated
- ☐ Thinking, "I can't deal with this"
- ☐ Loss of appetite for food, fun or sex
- ☐ Eating too much or too little
- ☐ Loss of sense of humor
- ☐ Little interest in personal appearance
- ☐ Loss of interest in other people
- ☐ Feeling everything is pointless
- ☐ Tearfulness
- ☐ Forgetfulness

If you checked off more than five boxes, you may already be suffering from stress. On pages 210–211, you will find expert advice on how to control stress now and in the future.

ELIMINATING STRESS

The findings of the Interheart study (see page 17) highlight how important it is to eliminate stress from your life. The study showed that psychological influences, including stress, account for almost a third of heart attacks, almost as high a proportion as smoking. But it also identified one positive psychological factor in the battle against stress and cardiovascular disease. People with a high "locus of control"— those who feel like they're in charge of their own destiny—have a 25 percent lower risk of heart attack than those who feel buffeted by random forces beyond their control. They are generally happier and less likely to become depressed. And if you adapt well to stress, you are 25 percent less likely to have a stroke. The good thing is that you can apply these findings to your own work or home life straightaway. For example:

- Recognize that in most situations you do have a choice, if only about how to react, and it is your own choices that largely determine what happens to you. So at times of uncertainty, repeat to yourself, "I have a choice."
- Counteract negative thinking. If you find yourself thinking, "There's nothing I can do about this," remember that there is usually some aspect of your situation that you can influence.
- Work at becoming more decisive and developing your problem-solving abilities.

Everyone reacts differently to stress. Some people take it in stride; others become tense, angry, irritable or tearful.

PANIC ATTACK

Acute feelings of panic can occur at any time, usually for no clear reason—and they put you at an increased risk of heart disease. British researchers, who found that people under 50 diagnosed with panic attacks or panic disorder were 38 percent more likely to have a heart attack and 44 percent more likely to develop heart disease than others. Risks were raised to a lesser extent in people over 50. Possible reasons include the effect of intense nervous activity on the heart and blood vessels.

In one doctor survey, 8.6 percent of primary-care patients said they had panic attacks. Overall, about one in ten North Americans gets occasional attacks—twice as many women as men. Symptoms include faintness, breathlessness, rapid heartbeat, chest pain, nausea, trembling and dizziness, accompanied by a feeling of deep anxiety or dread.

Eat healthily, sleep soundly and develop your sense of humor.

banishing stress in the long term

If you learn how to react well to situations that provoke sudden feelings of stress, you can devise a more long-term strategy for a stress-free existence.

- **Learn to relax** If you feel constantly under pressure, it is vital to carve out some time that is just for you, even if it is only half an hour a week. Progressive muscular relaxation can really help to alleviate the effects of stress on your body. It doesn't take long and it is really simple to do. Start by tensing the muscles in your feet, then relax. Then work your way up your body doing the same thing in sequence, from your feet to your head. Sometimes, it's only by experiencing muscle tension like this and letting it go that we become aware of just how much tension our bodies are retaining.

- **Let it out** If stress accumulates to such a degree that you feel like crying, take heart. Emotional tears are very different from the kind you produce when you're in pain or peeling an onion. Scientists think that a good cry actually clears out stress-related chemicals produced when we're under pressure. Some doctors speculate that this is why men, who cry less often, are more at risk of stress-related diseases than women.

- **Get high on exercise** Physical activity is one of the best stress-busters and, as explained in Step 7, one of the best exercise tools is easy to use and almost universally available: a staircase. When daily life starts getting you down, run up and down some stairs a couple of times or, if you can spare 10 minutes, go for a brisk walk around the block in the fresh air.

- **Eat healthily** A healthy diet helps to keep your immune system and metabolism functioning efficiently and protects you from the effects of stress.

- **Talk about it** Cultivate a support network. You might find it hard, but start sharing your feelings on a regular basis with at least one family member or trusted friend.

- **Control your use of imagery** Avoid using dramatic or overblown descriptions of problems in thoughts or speech, such as: "This job will be the death of me." We all do it, but exaggerating everyday difficulties increases their emotional intensity. If you say something like this inadvertently, counteract it with a strong dose of reality: "I'm still alive—so that's obviously nonsense."

- **Sleep soundly** Not only can stress interfere with your sleep, but not getting enough sleep can also add to your stress levels. See pages 224-27 for advice on how to make sure that you have a good sleep every night.

- **Create a sanctuary** Try to designate one place in your home that's truly "yours," where you can retreat when you need to get away from it all. Keep it free of clutter and make it as calming and restful as possible—with, for example, a favourite chair and a few objects you find visually pleasing.

- **Meditate or do yoga** When scientists measured the amount of atherosclerosis in the arteries of volunteers with high blood pressure, they found a significant reduction after nine months among those who'd learned to meditate (see page 213). And studies show that heart rates drop dramatically during a yoga class.

- **Get a view** Nature is a great stress-reliever. Studies have shown that patients experience less pain after surgery if they have a view of trees rather than a brick wall. And tests on students given a stressful task showed that their heart rates returned to normal faster when they gazed at a real fountain rather than at a digitally created image. Even photographs of restful scenes can help. So if the view from your window isn't great, try hanging a wonderful scenic photograph on the wall, or putting a plant or small vase of flowers in the place where you spend the most time.

- **Develop your sense of humor** Laughter is an excellent way to release tension from your body and help you to feel relaxed (see page 214).

dealing with anger

Anger can be a normal, healthy emotion that helps us to respond to a threatening situation. But it can also get out of control, and uncontrolled anger—sudden, intense fury—can actually provoke a heart attack or stroke. In fact, the risk of having a heart attack increases between nine and 14 times in the two hours after an angry episode.

The effect of anger was apparent in research involving more than a thousand people with implanted defibrillators—devices that automatically deliver a shock to the heart to control sudden, dangerous disturbances to heart rhythm. The researchers discovered that shocks were often needed following episodes of anger. An episode of moderate anger increased the risk of heart-rhythm abnormalities fourfold in the subsequent 30 minutes. Two hours later, people who got very angry had a risk ten times higher than that of people who remained calm.

LET IT OUT OR HOLD IT IN?

However you deal with it, intense anger is detrimental to health. Letting it out and holding it in can both do harm to your cardiovascular system.

A study that tracked 1,055 medical students for 36 years found that, by the age of 55, the men who showed the most anger were six times more likely to have had a heart attack and three times more likely to have developed any form of cardiovascular disease such as a stroke.

In another study involving 200 women, those who regularly displayed hostile attitudes, held in their anger and were more negative and self-conscious had a significantly higher risk of atherosclerosis in the carotid arteries supplying the brain ten years later.

STOP YOUR ANGER IN ITS TRACKS

First, figure out your pet peeves. What is it that really drives you crazy? Think in advance about how you might react differently next time. Recognize the warning signs of anger—rising irritation and a faster pulse or breathing rate, for example—and react to them by taking a break while you get things in perspective. Take deep breaths and give yourself a vital few seconds to release tension and avoid an impending explosion.

Regular exercise and relaxation will make you less prone to angry outbursts and more able to brush aside the little things that used to bother you. If you have a serious problem with anger, think about taking an anger-management course—it could improve your life, or even save it.

stay cool, stay calm

Relaxation techniques such as meditation are effective antidotes to stress, anger and unhappiness. There is no need to take a whole hour out of your day for a relaxation regime – a mere 15 minutes of quiet time will help you to unwind.

AN OASIS OF CALM

The notion of meditating may sound a little New-Age—like a fringe activity for hippies. In fact, it's something much more practical: In just 10 or 15 minutes, you can escape from the thoughts churning through your mind. Meditation and related activities, such as visualization, can be highly beneficial for people who feel anxious, hostile or angry. And the added beauty of these techniques is that you can practice them safely and easily at home, or maybe even in a quiet room in your workplace. Just follow these simple steps:

- **Comfort** Wear loose-fitting clothes and pick a quiet corner of your home (or an empty room at work) where you can relax. If you sit in an easy chair, don't slump—a straight posture helps breathing and keeps you mentally alert. Some people prefer to sit on the floor. Look at your watch or clock and decide to distract yourself for 10 or 15 minutes. Then choose a word or sound like "om" on which you can focus while you meditate.

- **Focus on breathing** You can close your eyes or keep them open, whichever feels most comfortable and helps you concentrate. Breathe deeply and repeat your chosen word or sound in your head every time you exhale, making sure you consciously direct your mind away from other thoughts and back to the sound. Keep everything else outside this little bubble of peace that encloses you. Focus only on the sound and on your rhythmic breathing; this will boost the oxygen supply to your body, reduce your heart rate and help you to relax. Your goal is to be awake and alert but not at all tense.

ESCAPE IN YOUR MIND

Or try visualization, which requires only your imagination. You simply sit, close your eyes and, using all your senses, conjure up a favourite scene—a beach, perhaps, where you can feel the sun on your face, see the seagulls swooping and taste the salty air. Just be there...until you unwind.

Escape in your mind ... conjure up a favorite scene.

have a **good laugh**

Laughter is a great way to relax and release tension, which would suggest that a lively sense of humor can boost your cardiovascular health. To test this hypothesis and investigate how laughter might protect arterial linings from the damaging effects of stress, cardiologist Michael Miller and his team at the University of Maryland School of Medicine asked healthy volunteers to watch comedy movies and studied the effects. They found that laughter relaxed their subjects' blood vessels and boosted blood flow by almost 25 percent—equivalent to the increases seen with light exercise or cholesterol-lowering drugs. Conversely, when the volunteers watched a tense dramatic film, their blood flow was reduced by more than a third—an effect similar to that caused by dwelling on bad memories or doing stressful mental math.

Intriguingly, laughter is also contagious; the saying "laugh and the world laughs with you" has an element of literal truth. When researchers scanned volunteers' brains while playing tapes of sounds that ranged from people laughing and whooping with triumph to screaming and retching, the positive sounds created much stronger responses. And the area of the brain that "lit up" in response to triumphant sounds or laughter was the same as the one involved in smiling, which suggests that the brain actually primes us to respond to other people's smiles by smiling back. This is also, of course, why producers of certain television sitcoms include canned laughter at the end of gags—they hope it will prompt a studio audience or viewers at home to laugh along too.

SECRETweapon

LAUGHTER YOGA

For those who want to combine getting in shape with having fun, there is an international laughter movement that runs "laughter yoga" classes. This gives you a chance to get together with other people and just laugh. It's an excellent aerobic workout, combining the physiological benefits of laughter with yogic breathing, which brings more oxygen to the body and brain. Laughter produces endorphins, making you feel good, reducing tension and relaxing your body. (See Resources, page 240, for advice on finding a class near you.)

Janine Capstack

"I'm a survivor"

In 2002, Janine Capstack experienced a day she will never forget. Janine was just 37 and recently divorced. She worked full-time as a personal assistant to a company finance director while looking after her two small boys. "I had just returned home after a trip," she says. "I did some laundry, made the children's supper and started to mow the lawn. Halfway through, I got a sudden sharp headache. I told the children to call my mom, went inside and collapsed on the bed."

Her mother telephoned the doctor, who told her to call 911. Doctors diagnosed a subarachnoid hemorrhage - bleeding inside the brain. Janine was paralyzed down her right side.

"I'm a believer in accepting what's happened and making the best of it. I'm a survivor."

"For what seemed like ages, my life was in ruins," she says. "I had to learn to walk and talk again." She was in rehabilitation for six months and still has some weakness on her right side.

Janine believes that her stroke was caused by the stress of her divorce and looking after the children on her own while working full-time. "I'd had high blood pressure since my younger son was two, but I never dreamed I was at risk of a stroke. I thought I was too young." As she recovered, Janine gave up smoking and made sure that the pace of her life slowed down. She now reads much more and takes naps in the afternoons. "Just half an hour, then I feel fine again. But I've got to sleep."

She also works only one day a week, and tries to walk as much as possible to relieve stress. Her diet is also healthier; she has cut out salt and eats plenty of vegetables.

Janine admits that it's been tough, but her advice to anyone in the same situation is to think positively. "I'm a believer in accepting what's happened and making the best of it. I'm a survivor."

THE BEST MEDICINE

When you're laughing, just like when you exercise, your blood pressure and heart rate rise slightly—but in the long term, regular laughter reduces blood pressure and boosts your immune system. And remarkable research from the University of Tsukuba in Japan has shown that laughter may even help to control blood-sugar levels in people with diabetes. Volunteers' blood-sugar levels were significantly lower after watching a comedy film than after a dry lecture.

Simply thinking about humor has been shown to have positive health benefits. The anticipation of watching a favourite comedy show reduces levels of stress hormones such as cortisol and increases levels of stress-relieving endorphins, the "feel-good" and pain-relieving hormones produced naturally by the body.

In fact, laughter gives your body something of a cardiovascular workout. When you laugh, your breathing rate rises, helping to transfer oxygen around the body—and around 400 different muscles are activated in the process, including abdominal and internal muscles that aren't involved in most exercise routines.

The positive effects of laughter were demonstrated in a small study of people in a cardiac rehabilitation program after a heart attack. A group of 24 patients watched a 30-minute comedy video each day for a year, and a similar group of 24 didn't. Only two of those who watched the video had another heart attack, compared with ten of the 24 people who didn't.

It seems that all human beings are born to find life fun, but that this capacity diminishes as we get older. On average, children laugh between 100 and 400 times daily, but once the stresses of adult life take hold, the frequency drops to between five and 15 times a day.

the power of happiness

Feelings of happiness, just like laughing or smiling, counteract the effects of stress. When scientists tested men and women taking part in a major study of heart disease risk, levels of cortisol were almost a third lower among people reporting their most happy moments during the day.

Regardless of your age, you can start feeling happier straightaway by making an effort to be more extroverted and energetic in your activities. According to psychologists, almost any active behavior—such as singing or dancing to music you hear on the radio—has a positive effect on your mood. And, like laughter, happiness is contagious. According to data gleaned from the massive Framingham Heart Study, which spanned three decades, happiness spreads from person to person. Analysis of the social networks of the inhabitants of Framingham, MA, revealed that the happiness of a friend living within a mile of you increases the likelihood of your own happiness by 25 percent.

SHARED PLEASURE

The effects of happiness are stronger between friends of the same sex and can be seen at three degrees of separation—your friend's friend's friend's happiness affects your own. And again, say researchers, "clusters of happiness result from the spread of happiness and not just a tendency for people to associate with similar individuals." Curiously, in this study, the influence of friends seems significantly greater than that of spouses or siblings. Having a happier partner increased subjects' happiness by only 8 percent, and a happier sibling by 14 percent—but a next-door neighbor who became happier boosted a person's chance of happiness by 34 percent.

What seems clear is that, in general, a key determinant of human happiness is the happiness of those around you. This accords with other research showing how emotions can be contagious, both in the short term ("service with a smile" really does make customers more cheerful) and over longer periods. Similarly, students living with a mildly depressed roommate are more likely to become depressed themselves. "People's happiness depends on the happiness of others with whom they are connected," the Framingham team concluded. Detailed

A FURRY FRIEND

The companionship of a pet may benefit your health in important ways by reducing stress levels. Studies have shown that pet owners have better than average survival rates following a heart attack, and a lower risk of succumbing to cardiovascular disease in the first place. And older people who own pets are generally healthier and happier than those who don't. According to researchers, having a dog does more for your heart than having a cat—dog owners in the study had lower than average blood-cholesterol and blood-pressure readings, possibly because of the extra exercise they get while taking their pets for walks.

analysis of the statistics from the happiness study demonstrates that each happy person you know increases the likelihood of your own happiness by 9 percent.

FIND A FRIEND ...

Unsurprisingly, other research indicates that the more friends people have, the more likely they are to be happy. When Britain's National Lottery commissioned a study to investigate happiness among lottery winners and others, it turned out that people who described themselves as "extremely satisfied" with life had twice as many friends as those who were "extremely dissatisfied." The optimum number of friends for happiness seems to be ten.

... AND LIVE LONGER

The number of friends you have may even affect how long you live. In one Australian study, conducted over ten years, people over 70 who had a strong network of friends lived longer than those with weaker social links. Other studies show that people with more friends are more likely to survive a heart attack, less likely to have a stroke and do better after being discharged from the hospital. Men who are less sociable have a greater cardiovascular risk, and score higher in blood tests for inflammation (see page 22).

MARRIED OR SINGLE?

While deaths from heart attacks and strokes are higher in unmarried than married men, having a close group of friends can protect you if you're single. As explained above, friends can have a powerful influence on your happiness—and your health. In one study, the health risks to men living alone were worse than those of people who smoked, while being married reduced mortality in men by 9 percent over a seven-year follow-up period—greater than the effect of not smoking. However, for married women, the risk of dying within seven years was reduced by only 2.9 percent compared with single women. Being divorced actually seems to protect women—but not men—against heart disease.

SECRETweapon

A HOT DRINK

If you are trying to make new friends, asking people to come over for coffee could have surprisingly successful results. If you want someone to warm to you, give him or her a hot drink, say scientists. In one study, volunteers who had just held a cup of hot coffee rated characters in a story as 11 percent "warmer" (more generous and caring) than they had just after holding a cup of iced coffee. Holding something warm also makes people feel warmer and more generous themselves since physical warmth promotes trust between people.

GENDER GAP

The fact that men are generally more reticent than women appears to increase their risk of cardiovascular problems. But what accounts for this phenomenon? One theory is that women are more likely to have close friends in whom they can confide, and therefore benefit more than men from external social support—so being married makes relatively little difference to their risk of heart disease or their mortality rates. In contrast, men are much more likely to confide primarily in their wives or partners than in friends, so being single puts them more at risk.

Another explanation for the gender gap is that, when it comes to health, being married affects men's behavior measurably more than women's. Single men— whether divorced, separated or never married—are much more likely to eat prepackaged meals than married men. They're also less likely to go for checkups and have a higher mortality rate from cardiovascular disease and other causes, whereas such differences are either not seen or appear to a lesser extent between single and married women.

HUG YOUR WAY TO HAPPINESS

A hug is good for your emotional health, and four hugs a day is also one of the ingredients of a happy marriage, according to a survey of 4,000 couples.

Couples who described themselves as happy or very happy were also likely to share at least two dinner dates and one breakfast in bed every month, as well as taking romantic walks and making romantic gestures. Other research has shown that hugs and physical displays of affection such as stroking or holding hands can reduce high blood pressure, speed up recovery from a heart attack, lower levels of the stress hormone cortisol and reduce the strain on the cardiovascular system caused by stress and anger.

Four hugs a day is one of the ingredients of a happy marriage.

mind over matter

The healthier you believe yourself to be, the less likely you are to die prematurely—no matter how healthy you actually are. One of the earliest studies to highlight this phenomenon used data from a survey of 7,000 older people in California in 1965, and compared their own reports on their health with mortality levels over the next nine years.

Men who initially reported their health as "poor" were more than twice as likely to have died as those who said their health was "excellent," even after the data had been adjusted to take account of age, physical health status, health practices, health relative to people of the same age, income, level of education, social and psychological factors. The outcome for women was even more startling. Women who saw themselves as being in poor health were more than five times as likely to die as those who thought they were healthy, irrespective of their actual health status.

Other research has demonstrated that men who believe themselves to be at lower-than-average risk of cardiovascular disease actually had a threefold lower risk of death from heart attacks and strokes over the following 15 years, even though almost half of them would have been classified medically as being at high or very high risk.

Are you an optimist? If so, you're lucky. Optimists have a powerfully beneficial effect on their own health.

POSITIVE THINKING

If you are an optimistic person, you're lucky. Optimists have a powerfully beneficial effect on their own health—and are much less likely than pessimists to die of cardiovascular disease, according to a study of older people in the Netherlands. Over a nine year follow-up period, those who reported high levels of optimism were 23 percent less likely to die of heart disease or stroke, and 55 percent less likely to die at all, than those with lower levels. By contrast, people who displayed a sense of hopelessness had a higher incidence of cardiovascular disease.

THE KEY TO SURVIVAL

A study that followed the fortunes of 96 men who had had a first heart attack revealed that having an optimistic outlook also reduced the chance of a further attack. The researchers kept a close eye on their subjects'

Joanna Cruddas

Finding a haven

In a corner of her city, Joanna Cruddas has found a haven from urban pressures. Two years ago, she was given a plot in a community garden, where she spends several hours a week during spring, summer and fall. Gardening is in Joanna's blood: Her aunt was a professional gardener and her parents were enthusiastic amateurs. "I remember, as a child, the immense satisfaction of weeding a flower bed, then watching the plants flourish, of sweeping leaves in the autumn and sitting in the first warmth of spring sun surrounded by daffodils."

Now in her fifties, she still experiences that contentment and finds gardening to be an antidote to hectic modern life. "Shutting the gate of the garden is shutting the gate on the outside world," she says. "Once I start to dig or plant, it becomes a totally absorbing relationship between me, the earth and the plants, and I lose all track of time."

Focusing on a simple task - what you have to cut back or tidy next - allows you to forget about your problems. Gardening is an excellent form of exercise, too. Weeding, digging and

"Once I start to dig, it becomes a totally absorbing relationship between me, the earth and the plants."

mowing all count as moderate physical activity, and energetic gardening for 10 minutes can burn 55 to 60 Cal. Weeding or pruning burns 300 Cal an hour, and digging 400 Cal. "There is nothing like raking leaves to get the heartbeat going," says Joanna. "For me, the best benefit has been in building upper-body strength. In this age of convenience, it's easy for muscles to weaken. Carrying watering cans, lifting and spreading compost - they've all made a huge difference to the strength of my spine and shoulders."

At the end of an afternoon's physical work, relaxing with a cold drink and being able to see the results of your exertion is wonderfully fulfilling, she says. "That's when I sit on my bench and plan what I'll do in the future, while enjoying the companionship of my neighboring gardeners."

moods and reactions to events. Over the following eight years, 15 of the 16 most pessimistic men had died of another heart attack—whereas, among the most optimistic group, 11 of 16 had survived.

THINK YOURSELF HEALTHY

Several scientific studies have found that it is perfectly possible to think yourself healthy. Psychologists who observed 84 female hotel workers found that, although the women were clearly getting plenty of exercise—each cleaned 15 rooms per day on average—most didn't count their work as exercise. Two-thirds claimed not to exercise regularly, and more than a third insisted that they got no exercise at all. The most amazing finding was that the workers' cardiovascular health, as measured by blood pressure, weight, body fat, BMI and waist-to-hip ratio, was related to how much exercise they *thought* they were getting—not how much they actually got.

The psychologists then went a step further. They took aside half of the hotel workers and spent an hour explaining to them how the amount of exercise they got from their jobs more than met the requirements of a healthy and active lifestyle. They also gave out fact sheets showing how many calories are burned by various cleaning activities. The other group of workers was given no such information.

Four weeks later, both groups were reassessed. Activity levels had not changed in either group, but those given information about the health benefits of their work now perceived themselves as doing more exercise—and they had become healthier, as well. They had lost weight, removed inches from their waist measurements, reduced their body fat, BMI and waist-to-hip ratios, and improved their blood pressure—simply as a result of being given the information and believing that they had a healthier lifestyle than they had formerly thought. The study is an especially compelling example of the power of positive thinking.

never stop learning

You may be aware that by continuing to be mentally active you can help stave off the decline in cognitive function that often accompanies the onset of late middle age, and reduce your risk of dementia. In fact, mental exercise, just like physical exercise, seems to be protective. But did you know that exercising your mental muscle may also help to stave off cardiovascular disease?

USE IT OR LOSE IT

Scientists know that people whose mental function declines as they get older have a higher risk of coronary artery disease. But until recently, it was not clear whether the same mechanism—atherosclerosis—underlies both heart attack risk and reduction in cognitive ability. Now researchers from Britain's University of Bristol have a possible answer.

They studied data from more than 11,000 people born in the United Kingdom in the early 1950s, whose intelligence was measured at the ages of seven, nine and 11 and who were followed into adulthood. Statistically, those with a lower IQ had a higher risk of future cardiovascular problems. However, the link between lower childhood intelligence and cardiovascular risk virtually disappeared when men and women stayed mentally active.

The study strongly suggests that keeping your brain agile in adulthood has a greater effect on your cardiovascular health than anything in your background, and is a further key to avoiding heart attacks and strokes. If you've always wanted to get a few more qualifications, learn a language or take some college courses, now you have an extra reason to give it a try.

Keeping your brain agile by giving it plenty to do could help stave off cardiovascular and cerebrovascular disease.

sleep well

The average amount of sleep that we get each night has fallen by around two hours over the past 40 years—not a good development for our cardiovascular systems. Adequate sleep is an important insurance against a range of risk factors including obesity, metabolic syndrome, diabetes and high blood pressure, and people who don't get enough sleep are more likely to develop atherosclerosis. In one study, scans showed calcified arteries—a measure of atherosclerosis—in almost one in three people who slept less than five hours per night, whereas getting just one more hour lowered the number of people affected to one in ten.

DON'T SKIMP ON SLEEP

Blood pressure and heart rate are typically at their lowest during sleep, and people who sleep less tend to have higher blood pressure.

Women who lose sleep are particularly at risk, with those who sleep five hours or less a night twice as likely to suffer from hypertension as women who sleep seven hours or more. Research findings from a study of the sleep patterns of about 10,000 people found that those who habitually slept five hours a night or less doubled their risk of dying from cardiovascular disease when compared with those who slept for seven hours or more. The bottom line is people who sleep well live longer.

THE MIDDLE WAY

In fact, sleeping too little and sleeping too much are both bad for the health of your cardiovascular system. Sleeping for five hours or less, or for nine hours or more, are both linked with a higher death rate from cardiovascular disease compared with sleeping for around seven hours a night. The results are so marked that, according to current scientific opinion, how long people sleep may be a key predictor of their heart-disease risk. The explanation may lie in the increased risks of diabetes and high blood pressure among people with very short or very long sleep-duration patterns.

Some people don't stay in bed long enough to get a decent night's sleep. For others, however, insomnia prevents them from getting the sleep they wish they could have. There are several patterns of sleeping difficulties:

- Not being able to fall asleep—maybe because you are too alert, worried, cold or hungry at bedtime.
- Being disturbed during the night— for example, by pain, noise or the need to go to the bathroom.
- Waking up too early in the morning and being unable to get back to sleep. This may be a symptom of depression, so if it happens frequently, it is worth mentioning to your doctor.

DAYTIME DOZE

Sleep disruption is particularly hazardous since it increases the levels of several blood-clotting factors, therefore raising the risk of blood clots. And if your sleep is regularly disturbed, the chances are that you will feel

SNORING

Often more than just a localized problem of the nose or throat, snoring may be linked to cardiovascular disease. If you snore, you are at risk of a condition called obstructive sleep apnea, in which the throat narrows to the point where you stop breathing. Typically, you give a loud snort, wake up and then start breathing again. This may happen repeatedly throughout the night, though sufferers are often unaware of it.

Both snoring and sleep apnea are more common in people who are overweight. This is a double-edged sword, since you are more likely to gain weight if your sleep is disturbed. Sleep apnea has also been linked with inflammation, insulin resistance (see page 30), abdominal fat and metabolic syndrome. It puts you at risk of cardiovascular disease and increases your chances of high blood pressure.

The good news is that measures to reduce metabolic syndrome—eating a healthier diet and getting more exercise, for example—also help to ease nighttime breathing disturbances. In severe cases, the snorer may be advised to wear a special mask in bed that keeps the airway open by gently pumping through a flow of air.

If think you may have sleep apnea, or even if you just snore a lot, talk to your doctor. You may need to be evaluated at a special sleep clinic. And don't forget that, if you don't snore but you share a bed with someone who does, you may be at greater risk of disturbed sleep than your partner (see page 198).

sleepy during the day. According to a large study of risk factors for cardiovascular disease, daytime sleepiness was associated with a 35 percent increased risk of cardiovascular disease in men and a 66 percent increase in women. It also increased the risk of heart failure by 49 percent among men and more than 50 percent in women. So it's worth taking time to find out the cause of your disturbed nights, especially if you are a woman.

SNOOZE ALERT

Nodding off when you sit down to read a newspaper or watch television could be a sign that you are at risk of a stroke. According to one study of 2,000 people, those who reported snoozing during the day when they didn't intend to fall asleep were more than twice as likely to have a stroke over the next two years as those who did not—and those who said this happened often had a risk four and a half times higher than normal. So

Snooze alert ... If you've developed a habit of unintentional daytime dozing, see your doctor for a checkup.

if you have developed a habit of unintentional daytime dozing, see your doctor for a checkup.

SLEEP SOLUTIONS

When you are lying awake exhausted but are still too alert to sleep, it can feel like insomnia is an insurmountable problem. In fact, for many people it is easily resolved—without a prescription. You just need to pay attention to what the experts call "sleep hygiene." Here are their recommendations for ensuring that you sleep soundly:

● Make sure your bedroom is dark, quiet and sufficiently warm, but not too warm—slightly cooler than your other living areas is ideal.
● Reserve your bedroom for sleep (and sex). Don't watch television or work in bed.
● Step up your daytime activity. Regular exercise, preferably in the fresh air, promotes nighttime sleep. If you are tired during the day or having trouble dropping off at night, try exercise in the late afternoon. About five or six hours after exercising, there is typically a slight fall in body temperature, which helps to promote sleep. Don't exercise in the two or three hours before bedtime though, or you may be too alert to drift off.
● Go to bed at the same time every night and get up at the same time every morning.
● Establish a consistent winding-down routine in the evenings so that you are properly relaxed by bedtime. Avoid stimulating television or movies and boisterous activities for at least two hours before bedtime.
● Avoid caffeinated drinks such as tea and coffee in the evenings. Don't smoke (nicotine is a stimulant) and limit your alcohol intake.
● Don't eat a huge meal late at night.
● Try herbal remedies to help you relax, like chamomile or valerian tea.

moving forward

The nine steps completed so far cover everything from knowledge and risk to diet, exercise and mental well-being, giving you most of the defenses you need to avoid heart attacks and strokes—not to mention live more energetically and contentedly. But there is one more step to follow, since the key to the overall plan is to keep all your self-defense strategies going so that they become a lifelong blueprint for health and happiness.

self-defense plan

STEP 10

ONCE YOU HAVE BEGUN TO DEVELOP YOUR PERSONAL PROTECTION PLAN AGAINST HEART DISEASE AND STROKES, YOU SHOULD SOON START TO EXPERIENCE SOME BENEFITS. BUT, TO BE EFFECTIVE IN THE LONG TERM, ANY LIFESTYLE CHANGES MUST BE SUSTAINED. HERE ARE SOME TACTICS THAT WILL HELP YOU TO REMAIN ACTIVE AND HEALTHY IN THE FUTURE.

Make your plan lifelong

● **I**f you have come this far in your quest to fend off heart disease and strokes, you will have absorbed a great deal of information. If you have also applied your discoveries to your own life, you should be feeling less stressed, more active and energetic, and generally happier.

It is important to take pleasure in your new healthy lifestyle—but it is equally important not to become complacent. It is all too easy in the first few weeks and months to let goals slip as your willpower weakens. Step 10 describes the tools you need to keep your plan going and to build in new, positive strategies for lifelong protection.

As you start to experience the benefits of cleaner arteries, reduced cholesterol and lower blood pressure, you will realize that they are a direct result of the well-informed choices you are making every day.

stay motivated

Keeping your goals and rewards at the front of your mind will help you to stay motivated. So remind yourself repeatedly of the benefits of your new lifestyle: You will continue to feel reenergized, healthier and stronger—and you will almost certainly live longer, too.

Make positive, specific and detailed plans about how you can achieve your aims. If you change one element of a carefully thought-out regime, make sure to substitute it with something else that provides equal benefits and is just as easy to organize. For example, if your local swimming pool closes, switch your regular Tuesday afternoon swim with friends to the pool at the nearest gym—or resolve to go bowling or skating with the same group instead. Don't put it off; make sure that you have something of equal value to do the very next week. Enlist the help of like-minded people to help you to stay on course.

MAKING PROGRESS

Motivation also relies on the ability to keep moving forward. Although you may have made some progress since starting to read this book, it is unlikely that you will have achieved all your goals to your total satisfaction. Maybe you've lost 10 lb, but you'd really like to lose another 10 lb. Or perhaps your resting pulse rate is still a few beats short of your target rate, or you could still afford to lose a few inches from your waist measurement. Keep going by breaking down larger goals into smaller ones. If you want to lose 10 lb, start by aiming to be 1 lb lighter by the end of the week or 3 lb lighter by the end of the month.

And you can always add new ingredients to the mix: new ways to cook healthily, new sports to keep you interested, new activities to pursue and new friends to make. That's all part of treating your plan as a lifelong recipe for health and enjoyment, a pursuit that never ends.

TACTICAL SUPPORTERS

Also, remember some of the useful tactics that make it easier to fulfill your aims: using the stairs rather than taking the elevator, eating breakfast, enjoying the sunshine. Think of music, olive oil, a glass of wine, yoga, laughter, chocolate, sleep and friendships. The sheer scope of this list shows that opportunities for boosting your health are everywhere. It may help to make a list of the tactics that you've found most helpful, or most fun, and put it up on the fridge or anywhere else where you will see it regularly. Don't forget to add to it. Part of the enjoyment of your plan is to make it a living, dynamic thing, so always be open to new ideas that could help you on the way.

Friends, laughter, sunshine, chocolate, music and many other elements of daily life can provide tactical support.

mind over matter

Believing in yourself will make it easier to maintain your new healthy lifestyle. The more confidence you have in your ability to exercise regularly, the more likely you are to enjoy it and the less likely you are to give up, say Canadian public health researchers who surveyed more than 5,000 people. The other key factor for success is motivation—or how much you intend to exercise. If you stay confident and motivated, chances are you will stay physically active.

take **control** of your destiny

As revealed in Step 9, optimists are less likely than pessimists to develop cardiovascular disease—and optimists generally feel more in control of their lives. If you think you need to develop a more positive mental approach, concentrate on the things you do well. The vital aspects are:

- **Focus** Try to keep your thoughts directed toward what you want, not what you don't want. Visualize yourself in elegant evening attire or in the jeans you've always wanted to wear, or on a beach with the kind of body you've always yearned for. Block out the reflection of the overweight person you spotted yesterday in a shop window. The sooner you focus on a positive goal, the sooner you can plan how to achieve it.
- **Self-confidence** Keep your mind on moving closer to your goals, rather than indulging in negative thinking. Dwell on what you have accomplished. Take time to write down your successes, however small. You've reached Step 10 of this book, for a start, which means you probably know a great deal more about heart attacks and strokes—and how to prevent them—than many of your friends and neighbors.
- **Attention to detail** To achieve any long-term goal, you need to work on the details. Breaking down big tasks into small steps makes them more manageable and allows you to follow a predetermined sequence, helping to avoid the procrastination that derails so many good plans.

DEALING WITH SETBACKS

Staying positive is even more crucial if you fail to achieve your immediate goals as soon as you had hoped. In many cases, people embark on a new health regime with the best of intentions, succeed for a while, then slip back into less healthy habits. This can often make the original problems even worse. Remember the warnings in Step 5 about yo-yo dieting?

Remind yourself that you're only human. By being aware that you are likely to encounter setbacks, and by anticipating the bad moments, you can plan ahead for those times when you are most vulnerable.

If you find yourself falling back into old habits, the first thing to do is think about your original motivation and assess whether it is still valid, and whether it can be strengthened and made more relevant.

Then, analyze your strategy to see whether the goals you have set yourself are as clear and specific as they should be. A vague desire to lose weight is not enough. You need well-defined goals, preferably written down. For example: Eat just one chocolate bar this week; have an extra portion of vegetables instead of potatoes with dinner on three nights of the week; go for a swim after work on Wednesday; take the kids for a bike ride on Saturday afternoon.

STOP AND THINK

Before you open that bag of chocolate-chip cookies or light another cigarette, stop and ask yourself why you are doing it. All too frequently, the underlying trigger that derails our good intentions is related in some way to stress. It may have been your clear intention to eat pieces of fruit rather than other, less healthy snacks all week, but you're under pressure at work and had a fight with your partner when you got home. The temptation is to think "Forget it," and tuck into those chocolates or down a double whiskey.

Feeling low or under pressure?
Use a stress-buster—call up a friend.

STRESS-BUSTERS

It is important to have some stress-beating tactics lined up to help you survive the times when you are most likely to give in to temptation. Decide in advance on a few actions you can take when you're feeling low or under pressure—for example, put on your coat and go for a short walk, dig in the garden, take a hot shower or have a self-indulgent soak in the bath. Call a close friend and have a good chat. You'll find that your mood will lift and the craving for oral gratification will subside. See Step 9 (page 210) for more advice on getting through the difficult times. Finally, if you do fall off the wagon, don't berate yourself. Remind yourself that you are making progress—you are a success. Give yourself encouragement, get back on to the program you have devised for yourself and focus on moving forward.

GET TO KNOW YOUR BODY

Maintaining commitment to your goals is easier if you understand, and can visualize, how your body will benefit from a healthier lifestyle—which is why each individual step in this book has been designed to contribute to that overall picture. For example, Step 5 explains that our bodies respond best to certain types of food, and Step 7 shows that, just like our hunter-gatherer forebearers, we are meant to be active; simply sitting down for too long makes blood fats collect in our arteries, causing plaque to build up over time (see page 146).

SECRETweapon

SET SMART GOALS

There is a formula used by businesspeople for setting out their aims that can help almost anyone be more effective in achieving success. When defining your own goals, make sure they are **SMART**, as exemplified below:

Specific "I will go to the gym for an hour at 4 pm every Thursday." (Not: "I'm planning to get more exercise.")

Measurable "I will substitute one portion of fruit for a chocolate bar every day this week." (Not: "I will eat more fruit from now on.") To find out if your goal is measurable, ask questions such as: "How much?" "How many?" "How will I know when it is accomplished?"

Achievable "I've decided to cut out fatty meats, burgers, fried foods and take-out." (Not: "I'm going to avoid all saturated fat.")

Realistic "I will take a deep breath whenever my partner irritates me." (Not: "I'm never going to argue again.")

Timely "I'm starting a diet on Monday and aiming to lose a few inches from my waist by May 1." (Not: "I want a 26-in (66-cm) waist.")

RED ALERTS

While you are making your body as healthy as possible to minimize the risk of a heart attack or stroke, don't forget to take account of those trigger factors that were outlined in Step 1. Rather than the steady drip of unhealthy factors that, over the long term, can lead to plaque, atherosclerosis and cardiovascular disease, triggers act in the short term to promote a heart attack or stroke in someone who is already susceptible.

In the context of a lifelong plan for a healthier lifestyle, you need to remind yourself repeatedly where the danger points lie so that you can work out how to avoid or counteract them:

- Acute stress caused by, for example, a failing business or highly challenging work deadline.
- Uncontrolled anger.

- A fat-laden, heavy meal.
- Extreme cold.
- Early mornings (especially Mondays).
- Commuting.
- Excessively loud noises.
- Irregular heavy exertion.
- Air pollution.
- Severe emotional upset.
- Death of a loved one.
- Binge drinking.
- Flu and other serious respiratory infections.

MORE COMPLEX THAN IT SEEMS

While the basic principles of avoiding cardiovascular disease are pretty straightforward—eat healthily, sleep well, avoid stress, get some regular

inside information
understanding risk

When considering potential health risks, it is easy to lose perspective. Let's say, for example, that you are worried about having a heart attack during intercourse. You read a newspaper story that says, "Heart attack risk for a healthy man doubles within two hours of having sex." That sounds like a big extra risk—newspapers tend to play on our fears. But the actual baseline risk is tiny. The odds of a man having a heart attack in any particular hour are about one in a million. Even if this figure is increased to two in a million, it is still not very high—in fact, the risk of an average man having a heart attack during sex is about the same as it would be if he were walking at 2–4 miles (about 3–6 km) per hour.

But are you much more vulnerable to a heart attack if you have had a previous attack? In that case, your baseline risk—or, in this case, what is called headline risk—increases tenfold and that, too, is doubled during or after sex. But that makes the odds a mere ten in a million without sex, and 20 in a million with sex—so the risk is still negligible.

And the more exercise you do (which includes sex), the less likely it becomes that you will have a heart attack at all, because your overall risk will go down as you get in shape.

This is just one example of why doctors distinguish absolute risk (the one, or ten, in a million) from relative risk (the twofold, or tenfold, increase). Relative risks make good newspaper headlines, but, as explained above, even a tenfold increase in risk may still represent a very small absolute risk. So, whenever you come across risk statistics, ask yourself whether the number in question refers to relative or absolute risk.

exercise and keep your weight within normal limits—the mechanics of just how to achieve this are much more complex. This book has tried to clear up the complexity and put forward an enormous variety of different suggestions for helping you to achieve your aims in ways that are most suitable for you.

In reading *Conquering Heart Attacks & Strokes*, you will also have gained a lot of information about "hidden" factors that can make a difference to your risk of both events—everything from the dangers of gum disease or living next to a noisy road, to the protective effects of friendship or watching comedies.

KNOWING YOURSELF

By now, you will be aware of which topics covered in this book are most relevant in your case—whether these are health factors that you need to deal with, or tactics for protecting yourself. It is worth making a note of these items now and refreshing the list in the months and years to come, because neither you nor your life circumstances will remain static.

HELPING OTHERS

If someone close to you is unfortunate enough to have a heart attack or stroke, after reading this book, you should be equipped with the knowledge to spot the signs and act decisively and quickly.

It is worth refreshing your memory from time to time about the crucial symptoms of heart attacks and strokes (see Step 2, pages 40–45). And if you can, sign up for a short first-aid course, so that you will know what to do if you ever need to resuscitate someone. Information about training courses is included in the Resources section (page 240).

social networks

Finally, never underestimate the important part that relationships with family, friends and even neighbors can play in helping to fend off cardiovascular disease. We are, after all, social animals—and supportive friendships have a much more crucial role in maintaining good health than most people acknowledge.

Take stress, for example. Many studies have demonstrated that chronic stress can take a serious physical toll, contributing to heart problems by raising blood pressure and increasing blood's tendency to clot. Having a few close friends—the kind to whom you can talk about anything—can relieve stress and mitigate its harmful effects on your body. Remember the research showing that happiness can spread among groups of friends (see page 217). Among the many remarkable findings from those studies, one startling discovery is that emotions like happiness are more closely influenced by our friends than by our partners or siblings.

OUR INFLUENCE ON OTHERS

The researchers also found that states of mind and behaviors can spread through social networks, almost like an infection. The explanation for this is not simply that individuals tend to make friends with people who have similar characteristics to themselves; rather, it shows that certain character traits can rub off on others. And the effects can be transmitted through three degrees of separation—your own friend is most likely to influence you, but your friend's friend has some effect, and even your friend's friend's friend can play a small role.

The conclusions that have been drawn from the happiness study include the contention that the same phenomenon can be applied to smoking behavior. The researchers suggest that there may even be a "three degrees of influence rule" that could also apply to depression, anxiety, loneliness, drinking, eating, exercise and other emotional states and health behaviors.

GETTING INVOLVED

Our bodies are responsive to a wide range of social relationships—even our interaction with our neighbors, who can exert a surprising influence on our happiness. The reason for this could be that, if we see our neighbors virtually every day, they contribute to our sense of belonging and support in the local community. This has a big impact on our sense of satisfaction with life.

So remember the benefits to your cardiovascular system of just being involved. Widen your social circle, talk to your neighbors, get involved in your community, volunteer with local groups, take up new hobbies and get together regularly with other people.

You can also enlist others in your efforts to adopt a healthier lifestyle. Tell people if you're trying to stop smoking; get their support when you want to lose weight; get a friend to join a gym with you, or go swimming, cycling or walking together.

relax in **heart-healthy style**

Here are some more ideas derived from recent research studies about how to improve the health of your cardiovascular system.

- **Choose joyful music.** Ultrasound scans of the blood vessels of people listening to various types of music showed that light music and love songs produced, on average, a 26 percent widening of the arteries compared with silence. Heavy-metal rock music had the opposite effect, making the participants anxious; such arterial narrowing could encourage atherosclerosis.
- **Listen to a calming CD.** A study of people living in retirement homes showed that listening to a CD designed to promote relaxation—such as a calming voice with ocean waves in the background—produced a 6.4 percent drop in blood pressure after four months using the 12-minute CD three times a week. In comparison, listening to a Mozart sonata for the same period dropped it just under 5 percent.
- **Try a Wii gaming console.** This involves holding a wireless remote control and swinging it like a golf club or tennis racket, while an onscreen computer-generated character carries out the movements. The Wii Fit—designed to strengthen muscles and develop posture, flexibility and aerobic capacity—comes with its own balance board which has sensors that detect your body's movements. Exercises encompass yoga, aerobics (running, stepping and hula-hooping), muscle toning (sit-ups and lunges) and improving balance (simulating ski slaloms and walking on a tightrope). Playing on a Wii is a highly social activity; family and friends can join in. A study in the *British Medical Journal* found that regular users of Wii Sports could burn up to 1,830 Cal a week and lose 27 lb a year.

Listen to calming music.

keep **going**

There is no point thinking of your new lifestyle as a quick fix—you need to keep it going. Celebrate your triumphs, sustain the successful changes you've made, modify those that aren't working and keep making small alterations and adaptations. Your plan shouldn't dominate your life, but neither should it disappear from it once you've finished this book; it should become a part of your daily routine, a continuing source of rejuvenation and enjoyment. So keep this book at hand and refresh your memory from time to time. Be determined to sustain your plan for as long as you live.

conclusions

You've seen throughout this book how simple lifestyle changes can slash your risk of cardiovascular disease and reduce your chances of succumbing to a heart attack or stroke. In fact, what *you* do can make as much difference to your risk as medical interventions—and often more.

So while your doctor can give you medication to treat high blood pressure, losing a little weight and cutting down the amount of salt you eat may be sufficient. You may think it's easier to pop a pill, but it's important to remember that all medications can have side effects. Eating more healthily has multiple benefits and definitely will not hurt you.

Similarly, the miracle of statin drugs is revolutionizing the lives of people with high cholesterol—but why not avoid the problem altogether? Eating less saturated fat helps to prevent plaque from ever building up in your arteries. And while technological developments can often save you if you suffer from a heart attack or stroke, why take the risk, when there are so many easy ways to avoid these hazards?

THE MULTIPLE BENEFITS OF LIVING WELL

This plan is not all about self-denial. A healthy life is also a full, enjoyable, interesting life. There are many ingredients in this plan that are positively self-indulgent, such as chocolate, comedy and companionship.

And that's a crucial factor about protective lifestyle measures which is often overlooked: Unlike drugs, they rarely have isolated results. While scientists can pinpoint individual chemicals with specific effects, such as resveratrol in red wine (see page 111), all natural foods are made up of a host of different ingredients that, together, can have effects far greater than the sum of their parts. Similarly, red wine is often enjoyed in a supportive, social setting, along with friends and good conversation.

So while each step outlined here is important, for optimal results make all of them a permanent part of your life. Don't allow yourself to become impossibly stressed at work; learn to relax or you risk undoing, for instance, the good effects of a healthy diet or losing excess weight.

THE SECRETS OF "HEALTHIER" NATIONS

What becomes very clear when looking at cultures around the world where lifestyle diseases like cardiovascular disease are less common is that while they often have a healthier diet, there are usually other protective "ingredients" in their lifestyle as well.

For example, green tea contains chemicals known as catechins and theanine that have been shown to have various positive effects. But the simple act of making the tea may be as beneficial. In one study of more than three thousand women aged 50 and over, those who regularly practiced the Japanese tea ceremony—an elaborate ritual for brewing and drinking green tea—lived longer than women who did not. It appears that the calming and relaxing effect of the ritual itself bestows benefits.

MORE THAN JUST FOOD

Often, protection cannot be nailed down to a single factor like food. No one knows if it was just the Paleolithic diet that protected our ancestors from cardiovascular disease, or also the activity that hunting and survival entailed. How much did tracking and chasing wild animals, or seeking and picking fruit and other produce, contribute?

Similarly, you've heard how the Mediterranean diet reduces people's risk of heart attacks and strokes (see pages 108–109). And you've seen that multiple ingredients of the typical Mediterranean diet—such as olive oil, fish, fruit, vegetables and red wine—all individually have protective effects. But the Mediterranean "package" also includes home-cooked food, leisurely meals with friends and family, laughter, siestas and sunshine.

Food in these countries is both important in itself and intimately interwoven with the joy of living, pleasant surroundings and good company. Contrast that with a hurried lunchtime sandwich that comes in a plastic wrapper, fast food and take-out meals laden with salt and fat, or microwavable meals eaten in front of the television.

THE WHOLE PACKAGE

So while it's good to find out just what works and how much, science can only provide a limited number of answers. What's really important is the whole package, because it represents a lifestyle—your lifestyle. And that's the ultimate message of *Conquering Heart Attacks and Strokes*.

Because, as you've seen, safeguarding yourself against heart attacks and strokes involves many diverse aspects, and there are so many different things that you can do to reduce your risk. The more that you can blend the ingredients together, the more likely you are to protect yourself not only from cardiovascular disease, but also from all the other damaging effects of lifestyle diseases. And the really great news is that, as well as being physically fit, you are likely to live not just a longer and healthier life, but a happier and more fulfilled one too.

resources

Alcoholics Anonymous General Service Office for North America
PO Box 459, New York, NY 10163
Tel: 212-870-3400 www.aa.org

International Taoist Tai Chi Society
134 D'Arcy Street, Toronto, ON M5T 1K3
Tel: 416-656-2110 www.taoist.org

Laughter Yoga International
A-001, Denzil Apartment, 3rd Cross Road, Lokhandwala Complex, Andheri (West), Mumbai—400053, India
Tel: +91-22-40109840 www.laughteryoga.org

Nicotine Anonymous
6333 East Mockingbird Lane, #147-817, Dallas, TX 75214
Tel: 1-877-879-6422 www.nicotine-anonymous.org

Nordic Walking North America
www.nordicwalkingna.com

Online cardiovascular risk calculators
www.qrisk.org
hp2010.nhlbihin.net/atpiii/calculator.asp

Online cholesterol converter
Convert between mg/dL and mmol/L for total cholesterol, HDL, LDL and triglycerides
www.onlineconversion.com/cholesterol.htm

USA

American Diabetes Association
1701 North Beauregard Street, Alexandria, VA 22311
Tel: 1-800-DIABETES www.diabetes.org

American Heart Association
7272 Greenville Avenue, Dallas, TX 75231
Tel: 1-800-242-8721 www.americanheart.org

American Institute of Stress
124 Park Avenue, Yonkers, NY 10703
Tel: 914-963-1200 www.stress.org

American Lung Association
1301 Pennsylvania Avenue, NW, Suite 800, Washington, DC 20004
Tel: 202 785 3355 www.lungusa.org

American Red Cross
www.redcross.org

American Sleep Apnea Association
16856 Eastern Avenue NW, Suite 203, Washington, DC 20012
Tel: 202-293-3650 www.sleepapnea.org

American Stroke Association
7272 Greenville Avenue, Dallas, TX 75231
Tel: 1-888-478-7653 www.strokeassociation.org

American Volkssport Association
Walking clubs across the USA
1001 Pat Booker Road, Suite 101, Universal City, TX 78148
Tel: 210-659-2112 www.ava.org

Mothers Against Drunk Driving
511 East John Carpenter Freeway, Suite 700, Irving, TX 75062
Tel: 1-800-438-6233 www.madd.org

National Institute on Alcohol Abuse and Alcoholism
5635 Fishers Lane, MSC 9304, Bethesda, MD 20892-9304
Tel: 301-443-3860 www.niaaa.nih.gov

ObesityInAmerica.org
An obesity information site created by the Endocrine Society and the Hormone Foundation
www.obesityinamerica.org

Canada

Canadian Council for Tobacco Control
192 Bank Street, Ottawa, ON K2P 1W8
Tel: 1-800-267-5234 www.cctc.ca

Canadian Diabetes Association
522 University Avenue, Suite 1400, Toronto, ON M5G 2R5
Tel: 1-800-226-8464 www.diabetes.ca

Canadian Obesity Network
Royal Alexandra Hospital, Room 102, Materials Management Centre
10240 Kingsway Avenue, Edmonton, AB T5H 3V9
Tel: 780-735-6764 www.obesitynetwork.ca

Canadian Lung Association
1750 Courtwood Crescent, Suite 300, Ottawa, ON K2C 2B5
Tel: 613-569-6411 www.lung.ca

Canadian Red Cross
170 Metcalfe Street, Suite 300, Ottawa, ON K2P 2P2
Tel: (613) 740-1900 www.redcross.ca

Canadian Sleep Society
4994 de Maisonneuve Boulevard West, Suite 103, Westmount, QC H3Z 3B9
Tel: 514-509-2113 www.css.to

Canadian Volkssport Federation
Walking clubs across Canada
PO Box 2668, Station D, Ottawa, ON K1P 5W7
Tel: 613-234-7333 www.walks.ca

Heart and Stroke Foundation of Canada
222 Queen Street, Suite 1402, Ottawa, ON K1P 5V9
Tel: 613-569-4361 heartandstroke.ca

Hypertension Canada
3780 14th Avenue, Markham, ON L3R 9Y5
Tel: 905-943-9400 www.hypertension.ca

MADD Canada
2010 Winston Park Drive, Suite 500, Oakville, ON L6H 5R7
Tel: 1-800-665-6233 www.madd.ca

ParticipACTION
2 Bloor Street East, Suite 1804, Toronto, ON M4W 1A8
Tel: 416-913-1511 www.participaction.ca

St. John Ambulance Canada
1900 City Park Drive, Suite 400, Ottawa, ON K1J 1A3
Tel: 613-236-7461 www.sja.ca

glossary

aerobic exercise the type that uses up oxygen, making you breathe faster. Aerobic exercise boosts cardiovascular fitness

aneurysm a ballooning out of an artery, due to weakness in its wall

angina chest pain due to coronary artery disease

angiogram an X-ray taken after injection of a special dye, to enable blood vessels to be seen

angioplasty widening a narrowed artery by threading a thin tube up from the groin and inflating a balloon at its tip

arteries the network of tubes carrying blood to supply oxygen and nutrients to body tissues

atherosclerosis the underlying process by which plaque is laid down in arteries in cardiovascular disease

BMI body mass index, a measure of body fat based on a person's height and weight

cardiac arrest when the heart stops beating and cannot pump blood. Without urgent treatment, the person will die

cerebrovascular disease cardiovascular disease affecting the arteries supplying the brain

cholesterol an important component of cell membranes and hormones; too much accumulating in the blood can lead to plaque formation

clotting blood coagulation important in wound healing, but can also be dangerous if it blocks an artery, causing a heart attack or stroke

coronary artery bypass graft replacing a diseased segment of coronary artery with a healthy blood vessel taken from elsewhere in the body

coronary artery disease cardiovascular disease affecting the arteries supplying the heart muscle

cortisol a hormone produced in the body at an increased level when someone is under physical or emotional stress

CPR cardiopulmonary resuscitation—attempts to restart the heart after cardiac arrest

decibel a measure of loudness; an increase of ten on the decibel scale means that a sound is ten *times* as loud

diabetes a disorder of insulin and blood sugar control

diastolic blood pressure the force on artery walls when the heart rests between beats

ECG (or EKG) electrocardiogram—a test of the electrical activity of the heart, often used to diagnose a heart attack

embolus (pl. emboli) a clump of some abnormal substance traveling around the bloodstream, such as a clot, globule of fat or air bubble

endorphins chemicals produced in the body that have painkilling and mood-enhancing effects

fibrinogen a protein involved in the blood's clotting response

gangrene death of part of the body, such as the cells of a toe

glucose the type of sugar produced from digestion of foods and used by the body for energy

gum disease infection and inflammation around the gums

hemorrhagic stroke stroke due to bleeding in an artery supplying the brain

HDL cholesterol high density lipoprotein cholesterol, the "good" fat that mops up LDL cholesterol from the bloodstream

heart attack blockage of one of the arteries supplying the heart muscle by a *clot* or *plaque*

hypertension medical term for high blood pressure

inflammation response of body tissues to injury, irritation or infection

insulin a hormone produced by the pancreas and important in the regulation of blood sugar

insulin resistance lowered ability of body cells to respond to insulin and metabolize blood sugar properly

ischemia reduced blood flow to a part of the body, resulting in damage to the tissues

ischemic stroke stroke due to a blood clot in an artery supplying the brain

LDL cholesterol low-density lipoprotein cholesterol—the "bad" fat that may accumulate in the bloodstream and promote plaque formation

lipids fats in the blood

metabolic syndrome a cluster of risk factors including abnormal blood fats, abdominal obesity, high blood pressure and disturbances in blood sugar control

myocardial infarction medical term for a heart attack

omega 3 fatty acids essential fatty acids found in oily fish and some plants

omega 6 fatty acids essential fatty acids found in processed vegetable oils

pedometer a device for counting how many steps someone takes

periodontal disease medical term for gum disease

peripheral vascular disease atherosclerosis affecting the arteries in the legs, causing a cramping pain when walking

placebo a pill or other treatment that has no active ingredient

plaque the fatty deposits laid down in arterial walls that are responsible for cardiovascular disease

platelets cells involved in blood's clotting response

potassium chemical in blood that balances the effect of sodium (salt)

refined carbohydrates starchy foods that have been heavily processed and are therefore low in nutrients—for example, white flour, white bread, white rice and pasta

saturated fats the type found in animal products, typically solid at room temperature

sedentary lifestyle one involving minimal activity, such as sitting at a desk all day

sleep apnea episodes of interrupted breathing during sleep, often associated with heavy snoring

sodium part of a salt molecule (sodium chloride); may be used on labels to indicate salt content

statins a type of cholesterol-lowering drug

stent a tiny tube left inside an artery to hold it open, often used to relieve coronary artery disease

systolic blood pressure the force on artery walls when the heart contracts to pump blood

thrombolytic therapy treatment with clot-busting drugs to try to relieve a heart attack or stroke

trans fats artificial, processed fats that behave like saturated fats in the body

transient ischemic attack (TIA) temporary interruption of blood supply to a part of the brain, or a "mini-stroke"

unsaturated fats the type found in fish and plants, typically liquid at room temperature

unstable angina severe angina symptoms not relieved by rest that may be mistaken for a heart attack

index

canned and frozen 35

portion sizes 109

potassium-rich 98

G

gangrene 20

gardening 79, 221

garlic 111, 115

garlic supplements 191

gastric banding 123

gender gap 219

getting up in the morning 42

ghrelin 133

gingivitis 177

glucose 30, 144

   see also blood sugar

glucose intolerance 30, 31, 134

glucose metabolism 145

glycogen 163

grapeseed extract 111

green tea 111, 121, 239

gum disease 14, 29, 68, 79, 84, 176-177

   dental hygiene 29, 68, 176, 177

   warning signs 177

gyms 151, 152, 157, 164, 165-166

H

hand washing 190

happiness 34, 79, 216-219, 236

   questionnaire 77

heart 13, 15, 37, 145

   arrhythmias 25, 37, 43, 53, 175, 198

   blood supply, interruption of 38, 40

Heart and Stroke Foundation of Canada 17, 45, 48, 50, 178, 241

heart attacks

causes 19-20, 22, 26, 40

diagnosis 52

diet and 105, 106, 107, 111

emergency action 37, 41, 47, 48-51

first-time heart attacks 17

hospital treatment 43, 52-54

medications 57

myths 38

peak times for 42, 187, 188, 206, 207

recovery and rehabilitation 40, 57-58

risk factors 13, 17, 18, 22, 23, 26, 27, 32, 58, 59, 64, 68, 175, 176, 192, 203, 205, 207, 208, 212

stress and 205, 207, 208

symptoms 41

triggers 24-25

heart rate 145, 157, 211

heatstroke 194-195

heavy metal toxicity 200

hemorrhagic strokes 24, 44, 55, 56, 204

heparin 53

high blood pressure 13, 14, 17, 19, 26, 64, 204

and aneurysm 20

benefits of exercise 28, 42, 145

cardiovascular risk 64

and diabetes 30

and heart disease 26

lowering 97, 98, 105, 110, 111, 145, 170, 174, 193

medications 57

and memory impairment 24

sleep deprivation and 224

stress and 204

and strokes 24, 26, 58

toxic chemicals and 200

homocysteine 32, 34, 106, 107, 108

understanding 234

unhealthy lifestyle choices 17

see also Interheart study

and under cardiovascular disease;
  diabetes; heart attacks; strokes

or specific risks, i.e. alcohol, stress

rowing 157

running 154, 157

S

salt 64, 71, 84, 85, 97-98

sedentary lifestyle 65, 85, 137, 146-147

selenium 200

self-defense plan

  creating 78-91

  danger signs, recognizing and taking
    action 36-61

  diet 92-115

  exercise 140-171

  goals and rewards 34, 90, 182, 229,
    230, 231, 233

  hazards, combating 172-201

  lifelong protection 228-237

  lifestyle changes 62-77

  motivation, maintaining 228-230,
    231, 232

  personal risk assessment 62-77

  staying positive 231-233

  understanding heart attacks and strokes
    12-35

  weight management 116-139

serotonin 227

sexual relations 61, 234

sibutramine 123

singing 170

single people 218, 219

skipping 169

sleep 145, 211, 224-227

  daytime sleepiness 225-226

  insomnia 225, 227

  questionnaire 74-75

  risk factors for heart attacks and strokes
    88

sleep hygiene 227

  too much/too little sleep 88, 133, 224, 225

sleep apnea 225

slurred speech 25, 45

smoking 13, 17, 19, 58, 64, 68, 82, 87, 173,
    178-186, 236

  and aneurysm 20

  cravings 184, 185, 186

  harm done by 178

  low-tar cigarettes 179

  quitting 84, 180-186, 241

    health improvements after 185

    nicotine-withdrawal symptoms 180

    therapies and medications 181

  secondhand smoke 178

snack foods 85, 90, 97, 99, 125,
    130-131, 132

snoring 14, 198, 225

soccer 157, 164

  watching 27

sodium *see* salt

soy 107, 121

stairs, climbing 85, 162, 167, 211

stanols 103

statins 27, 34, 82, 101, 238

sterols 103

stomach stapling 123

stress 19, 64, 203-211

  dealing with 145, 206-207, 209, 210-211

  effects of 34, 203-204, 235-236

radionuclide scans 29

theanine 239

thrombocytosis 20

thrombolytic drugs 38, 47, 53-54, 55-56, 69

thrombosis *see* blood clots

toxic chemicals 200-201

traffic noise 198, 199

transient ischemic attack (TIA) 25, 30-40, 56

TrekDesk 146

trigger factors 24-25, 233-234

triglycerides 23, 30, 100-101, 105, 121

troponin 52

tryptophan 227

V

veins 15

viral infections 19

visualization 126, 213, 231, 233

vitamin C 21, 23, 108, 109

vitamin D 192-194

vitamin E 109, 121

W

waist measurement 67, 81, 118, 120, 139, 201

waist-to-hip ratio (WHR) 67, 118, 120, 179

walking 65, 125, 143, 149, 152, 153, 154, 164-165, 171, 191

dog walking 169, 217

Nordic walking 153, 169

walking clubs 149, 168-169

warfarin 56

warm, keeping 187

weight gain

after quitting smoking 186

benefits of exercise 19, 34

see also obesity

weight, losing 116-139

crash diets 124, 126

exercise 134-135, 139, 153, 156

food diary 124, 130

goal setting 34, 90, 127, 139, 232

doctor's help, enlisting 122-123

healthy eating plan 128-129

meals

savoring 132-133

scheduling 130

medication aids 122-123

motivation 119, 120

portion sizes 130, 131, 132

relaxation techniques, using 126

surgical means 123

sustaining weight loss 129, 139

top tips 125, 132

weighing yourself 138-139

willpower 129, 130

yo-yo dieting 126

weight training *see* isometric exercise

white blood cells 22

whole grain foods 96, 100, 101, 128

Wii gaming console 237

women, and heart disease 38, 40, 41, 64, 67, 101, 107

World Health Organization 8

X,Y,Z

Xenical 122-123

yoga 126, 170, 211

zinc deficiency 200

Zyban 181

Project Staff

Project Editor Jesse Corbeil

Writer Sheena Meredith, MB BS

Medical Consultants
Dr. Graham Jackson, FRCP, FESC, FACC; Dr. Mark Berner, MD, CCFP (EM), FCFP

Proofreader Madeline Coleman

Senior Designer Andrée Payette

Designer Chris A. Cant

Cover Designers George McKeon, Andrée Payette

Reader's Digest Association (Canada) ULC

Manager, English Book Editorial
Pamela Johnson

Vice-President, Editorial
Robert Goyette

The Reader's Digest Association, Inc.

President and Chief Executive Officer Tom Williams

Executive Vice President, RDA and President, Lifestyle Communities Suzanne Grimes

Executive Vice President, RDA and President, Reader's Digest Community Dan Lagani

Executive Vice President, RDA and President, Allrecipes.com Lisa Sharples

Executive Vice President, RDA and President, Europe Dawn Zier

Library and Archives Canada Cataloguing in Publication
Conquering heart attacks and strokes : your 10 step self-defense plan / the editors at Reader's Digest.
Includes index.
ISBN 978-1-55475-074-0
1. Heart--Diseases--Prevention. 2. Cardiovascular system--Diseases--Prevention.
I. Reader's Digest Association (Canada)
RC672.C6 2012   616.1'205   C2011-901034-8

We are committed both to the quality of our products and the service we provide to our customers. If you have any comments about the content of this book, write to
Book Editor, Reader's Digest Association (Canada) ULC,
1100, René-Lévesque Blvd. W., Montreal QC H3B 5H5

To order copies of **Conquering Heart Attacks and Strokes**, visit us at our online store:
www.rd.com in the US
www.readersdigest.ca in Canada

Note to Readers

The information in this book should not be substituted for, or used to alter, medical therapy without your doctor's advice. For a specific health problem, consult your physician for guidance. The mention of any products, retail businesses or Web sites in this book does not imply or constitute an endorsement by the authors or by The Reader's Digest Association Inc. or by Reader's Digest Association (Canada) ULC.